BRAIN DEATH

What is Brain Death?
At what point does a human life begin or end?

Criteria and tests for death have changed throughout history. Recent advances in medicine, particularly in the areas of resuscitation, mechanical ventilation and cardiac pacemakers, have posed great philosophical and practical problems for traditional concepts of death and their associated criteria and tests. The concept of brain death, formulated to deal with practical decisions that have to be made in deciding whether a person is dead or alive, has been subdivided by some into whole-brain death, brain stem death and neocortical death, yet others do not adhere to any formulation of brain death whatsoever.

Thomas Russell presents an entirely new concept of death, viewing death as death of the organism as a whole and answering the question "what is death?" with an examination of what constitutes life. Drawing on philosophical arguments, Russell argues that all current concepts of brain death are conceptually inadequate but a new concept of death, applicable to all living entities, can encompass the traditional criteria and tests for death and does not entail any significant operational changes in the way in which death is diagnosed. From an historical review and examination of current concepts of death, Russell considers key topics including: different brain states, conditions for life, biological concepts, and the moment of death. Arguing that all current concepts of brain death are conceptually inadequate, *Brain Death* offers invaluable new insights for those researching or studying across areas of medical ethics, applied ethics, death studies and the philosophy of science.

This book is dedicated to Kirsty

ASHGATE NEW CRITICAL THINKING IN PHILOSOPHY

The *Ashgate New Critical Thinking in Philosophy* series aims to bring high quality research monograph publishing back into focus for authors, the international library market, and student, academic and research readers. Headed by an international editorial advisory board of acclaimed scholars from across the philosophical spectrum, this new monograph series presents cutting-edge research from established as well as exciting new authors in the field; spans the breadth of philosophy and related disciplinary and interdisciplinary perspectives; and takes contemporary philosophical research into new directions and debate.

Series Editorial Board:

Professor David Cooper, University of Durham, UK
Professor Peter Lipton, University of Cambridge, UK
Professor Sean Sayers, University of Kent at Canterbury, UK
Dr Simon Critchley, University of Essex, UK
Dr Simon Glendinning, University of Reading, UK
Professor Paul Helm, King's College London, UK
Dr David Lamb, University of Birmingham, UK
Professor Stephen Mulhall, University of Oxford, UK
Professor Greg McCulloch, University of Birmingham, UK
Professor Ernest Sosa, Brown University, Rhode Island, USA
Professor John Post, Vanderbilt University, Nashville, USA
Professor Alan Goldman, University of Miami, Florida, USA
Professor Joseph Friggieri, University of Malta, Malta
Professor Graham Priest, University of Queensland, Brisbane, Australia
Professor Moira Gatens, University of Sydney, Australia
Professor Alan Musgrave, University of Otago, New Zealand

Brain Death

Philosophical concepts and problems

TOM RUSSELL BSC, MB CHB, PHD, FRCS (EDIN), FRCS (GLAS)
Consultant Neurosurgeon
Lothian University Hospitals NHS Trust
Edinburgh, Scotland

Part-time Senior Lecturer
University of Edinburgh
Edinburgh, Scotland

Honorary Lecturer
Centre for Philosophy and Health Care
School of Health Science
University of Wales, Swansea, Wales

Ashgate

Aldershot • Burlington USA • Singapore • Sydney

© Tom Russell 2000

All rights reserved. No part of this publication may be reproduced, stored in a retrieval system, or transmitted in any form or by any means, electronic, mechanical, photocopying, recording or otherwise without the prior permission of the publisher.

Published by
Ashgate Publishing Ltd
Gower House
Croft Road
Aldershot
Hants GU11 3HR
England

Ashgate Publishing Company
131 Main Street
Burlington
Vermont 05401
USA

Ashgate website: http://www.ashgate.com

British Library Cataloguing in Publication Data
Russell, Tom
　　Brain death : philosophical concepts and problems. - (Ashgate new critical thinking in philosophy)
　　1. Brain death - Moral and ethical aspects 2. Death - Proof and certification - Moral and ethical aspects
　　I. Title
　　174.2'4

Library of Congress Cataloging-in-Publication Data
Russell, Tom, 1950-
　　Brain death : philosophical concepts and problems / Tom Russell.
　　　p. cm. -- (Ashgate new critical thinking in philosophy series)
　　Includes bibliographical references and index.
　　ISBN 0-7546-1210-4 (hardcover)
　　1. Death. I. Title. II. Series.

BD444.R87 2000
128'.5--dc21　　　　　　　　　　　　　　　　　　　　　　　　99-055603

ISBN 0 7546 1210 4

Printed and bound by Athenaeum Press, Ltd.,
Gateshead, Tyne & Wear.

Contents

1	Introduction and Historical Review	1
2	Current Concepts of Death and Brain Death	17
3	Is There a Difference Between Those Declared "Brain Dead" and Those in Persistent Vegetative State or Other Abnormal Brain States?	39
4	Reasons for Rejection of the Present Concepts of Death	59
5	Consideration of Different Brain States in Relation to Different Concepts of Death	75
6	Can There Be Necessary and Sufficient Conditions for Life?	89
7	Justification for the Adoption of a Biological Concept of Death	107
8	Does Anything that Contributes to Homeostasis Count Toward Homeostasis?	121
9	Is Brain Death Necessary and Sufficient for Death?	135
10	When does Death Occur?	147
11	Operational Changes as a Result of the Suggested Concept of Death	159
Index		179

"At what 'point' does a human life begin or end? The Darwinian perspective lets us see with unmistakable clarity why there is no hope at all of *discovering* a telltale mark, a saltation in life's processes that 'counts'. We need to draw lines; we need definitions of life and death for many moral purposes. The layers of pearly dogma that build up in defence around these fundamentally arbitrary attempts are familiar, and in never-ending need of repair."

Daniel C. Dennett. *Darwin's dangerous idea.* p. 513

1 Introduction and Historical Review

"Be absolute for death; either death or life"
Shakespeare *Measure for Measure*

Controversies over the Definition and Diagnosis of Death

It is widely believed that prior to the introduction of modern machines and medicine that there was a consensus that death occurred when the heart stopped beating and breathing ceased. I would suggest that this was true within limitations, but even if it were accepted as true, many important questions would remain unanswered:
- Were the heartbeat and breathing defined as constituting life itself or were they merely physiological indicators that life was present?
- Which of the two was more important?
- Were there any other vital events?
- What tests, if any, could be used to determine whether or not these other vital events had ceased?
- What was the connection between the death of an organism as a whole and the death of its discrete, separate parts?
- What was the relation between the end of physical vitality and personal existence?

All these issues have remained controversial to the present day.

Death in Antiquity

The combined observations of doctors, soldiers, butchers and executioners led most ancient societies to the conclusion that an organism's body parts did not always die simultaneously and that the normal functioning of certain specific organs was crucial for the continued existence of the organism as a whole. Classical Greek physicians held that death could begin in lungs, brain or heart but that the heart alone was the seat of life. They believed that the heart created the vital spirits that constituted the essence of life; thus, the heartbeat alone distinguished between the living and the dead. Breathing merely regulated the heat of the heart (Weiner,

1968; Acknerknecht, 1968). The brain did have a vital role. Hippocrates located reason, sensation and motion in the brain; a view shared by the anatomists of Alexandria and Galen. The early Church even localised specific mental faculties in specific ventricles of the brain (Bynum, Browne and Porter, 1981). However, the heartbeat remained the sole indicator of life and death.

This view, however, was not universal and in the Hebrew tradition, *ruach* or breath was primary, often defined as life itself. This view remained a strong influence in Christian thought as well, at least through the Middle Ages (Rosner and Bleich, 1979a). Even within Judaism the role of breath was not completely unchallenged, and a minority of Talmudic sages accepted the heartbeat as a valid alternative indicator of life and death (Rosner and Bleich, 1979b). Even less popular was the view of Maimonides, a twelfth century rabbi and physician, who asserted the vital significance of the head. He considered a decapitated body dead, even if it still moved, because its motions lacked the central direction that presumably indicated the guidance of a soul (Rosner and Bleich, 1979c). Thus, a variety of classical traditions recognised certain organs as crucial to the life of the organism as a whole, yet there was much disagreement over which organ and functions were vital and why they were so.

Different classical and medieval physicians not only differed in their definitions of life and their views on the physiological indicators that signified that life had ended; they also recognised cases in which the attempt to apply their definitions and indicators resulted in diagnostic errors. "So uncertain is men's judgement, that they cannot determine death itself" wrote Pliny. Galen listed hysteria, asphyxia, coma and catalepsy among the conditions he thought could suspend all signs of life for weeks without precluding recovery (Stevenson, 1975; Winslow 1746a). St Augustine knew a monk (aptly named Restitutus) who could suspend his own heartbeat (Augustine, 1972). Despite the centrality of breath in the Jewish tradition, Maimonides and Raashi both considered it possible to survive protracted drowning. The Bible credited Elijah with restoring breath to a corpse (Rosner and Bleich, 1979d). Ancient Egyptians and Romans both produced such volatile caustics as sal ammoniac and spirit of hartshorn, capable of restoring the vital functions in cases of syncope (Grier, 1937; Stevenson, 1975). Thus, even the absence of heartbeats and breathing did not always mean death.

However, it must be remembered that the diagnosis of death was not usually a clinical responsibility for the classical doctor due to Hippocratic medical ethics and its prohibition of medical treatment for terminal patients. The doctor's duty was to forecast an impending demise and then withdraw from the case and not to remain in attendance long enough to diagnose or certify actual death (Pernick, 1985a). Thus, when classical and medieval physicians spoke of the *proprietates mortis* or "the signs of death", they did not mention heartbeats, pulse or breath but repeated the portrait of impending death described in Hippocrates' Prognostikon (Robbins, 1970). Then, as now, the "signs of death" indicated when the doctor's job was finished, but for classical physicians these "signs" did not mean that the patient was actually dead. For most of Western history, the actual diagnosis of death has been primarily a non-medical function.

Various classical texts indicate practices employed to protect against erroneous diagnoses. The Talmud, for example, records that ancient Jewish custom was to visit a corpse in its crypt for three days after death to check for renewed vital signs (Rosner and Bleich, 1979e). During major epidemics, like the Black Death of 1348 and succeeding plague outbreaks, when such careful precautions were unsafe and impractical, the popular dread of being buried alive rivalled the terror of the disease itself (Winslow, 1746b). Thus, from the very beginning of Western history, defining and diagnosing death has proved both perplexing and controversial.

Death from 1740 to 1850

Death was never easy to define or diagnose, yet some historical periods demonstrated far more discomfort over these uncertainties than did others. One era of particularly intense concern began about 1740 and lasted through the middle of the next century or longer as the scientific, social and ethical effects of the Enlightenment combined to render the boundary between life and death frighteningly indistinct.

In the mid-seventeenth century, the Papal physician Paulus Zacchias had written that no sign prior to the start of putrefaction could reliably distinguish the dead from the living (Lancisi, 1971a; Garrison, 1929; Tebb and Vollum, 1905a), but it was not until the following century that such comments evoked much concern. In 1740, the eminent Franco-Danish anatomist Jacque Benigne Winslow published a Latin dissertation on "The uncertainty of the signs of death and the danger of precipitate interments and dissections" (Winslow, 1740). This was reprinted and published in French, Italian, Swedish and German and within two decades the whole of Europe was aware of the uncertainty of death. By 1850, the books and articles on the subject could be counted in the hundreds (Tebb and Vollum, 1905b). Dunglison's (1833a) pioneering medical dictionary agreed that "the only certain sign of real death is the commencement of putrefaction" an opinion shared by others (Hawes, 1780; Symonds, 1836; Orfila, 1818), while yet others doubted that even incipient decomposition could be distinguished reliably from such diseases as gangrene (Kite, 1788; Colhoun, 1823; Snart, 1824; Capron, 1980). The most dramatic result of physicians' lack of confidence in diagnosing death was the public panic over "premature burials"; this, in turn, was reflected in literature such as Edgar Allen Poe's "Fall of the House of Usher" and "The premature burial".

The reason for this doubt about the ability of the medical profession to distinguish the living from the dead was due to the discovery of artificial respiration. The pioneering works appeared in Paris in 1740 (Reaumur, 1740; Winslow 1740). These techniques spread rapidly, and in 1780 Hawes (1780) used the records of the London Society (a society set up to teach resuscitation methods) to prove that nothing short of putrefaction could distinguish death from life (Lee, 1972). Resuscitation measures at this time included measures to revive circulation as well as respiration but electric shock dominated the research and the first human case was reported in 1774 (Schechter, 1971; Kite, 1788b; Smith, 1821; Philip, 1834; Jellinek, 1947). Mary Shelley's account of "Dr Frankenstein" in 1818 dramatised both the ethical issues and the uncertainties about the distinctions between life and death. The introduction of inhalation anaesthesia in 1846 added further to the confusion (Stevenson, 1975; Pernick, 1985b). More controversial were those states of suspended animation deemed psychological or idiopathic, *e.g.* catalepsy, ecstasy and trance. In Paris in the 1780s, Franz Anton Mesmer induced in his followers a trance state he attributed to "animal magnetism". Mesmerism not only produced apparent death, by 1785 it was also claimed to have restored the dead to life (Darnton, 1968; Braid, 1850).

This increase in the number of death-like states seemed to require one of two possible responses. The fact that apparently unconscious, breathless and pulseless bodies could be revived might mean that these physiological functions were not essential to life. At least one member of the medical profession took this view (Schrock, 1835). If this was the case, then these functions could no longer be used as the criteria of death: new indicators and, perhaps, a new definition of death would be needed. The other possible response is that the vital functions never really stopped during such cases. Perhaps they really continued but at a level below the sensitivity threshold of the available methods of detection. In that case, all that was needed was better diagnostic testing without any change in indicators or definition of death. This latter view gained wide medical acceptance in the 1830s and 1840s and the solution to the problem was simply to devise more sensitive and reliable tests to detect these functions. The search for such procedures filled the literature and fell naturally into two groups. The tests for respiration included methods such as holding a candle, mirror or feather to the nose (Lancisi, 1971b; Tebb and Vollum, 1905c; Winslow, 1746c), submerging the body and watching for bubbles (Snart, 1824b), putting a bowl of liquid on the chest (See, 1880), using the new technique of auscultation with the recently invented stethoscope (Forbes *et al*, 1845) and holding an hygrometer to the nose (Snart, 1824b). Tests for circulation ranged from feeling the pulse manually or listening with the stethoscope (Littel, 1847) (although agreement about the latter was not universal (Kesteven, 1855)), to opening an artery (Snart, 1824b). Coldness signified the loss of "vital heat" (Smith, 1827; Ackerknecht, 1968b; Schrock, 1835b).

Failure to respond to artificial respiration soon gained acceptance as a (partly tautological) criterion of death. Likewise, failure to twitch in response to electrical resuscitation seemed useful as a test for loss of neuromuscular function. This distant predecessor of the flat brainwave test was first suggested by Charles Kite in 1788 (Kite, 1788b). Unsuccessful use of other revival techniques, from smelling salts (Snart, 1824b) to blowing a trumpet in the ears (Ackerknecht, 1968b) also were on the list of death tests suggested and used.

Each of these and many more had their advocates but only rigor mortis and putrefaction won any general acceptance, and even these were widely challenged, as already indicated. The response was to search for even more signs and tests. The eighteenth century Scottish physician William Cullen offered one based on the neurophysiology of Haller. Cullen concluded,

> "life does not immediately cease upon the cessation of the action of the lungs and the heart. The living state of animals does not consist in that alone, but especially depends upon a certain condition in the nerves... by which they are sensible and irritable. It is this condition, therefore, which may be properly called the vital principle in animals". (Cullen, 1784)

In addition to neuromuscular potential, another capacity of living beings that seemed unique and not reducible to eighteenth century laws of mechanics was their power to resist the physical forces of entropy and decay. Thus, Georg Stahl concluded that a body's ability to stave off putrefaction proved that it was still alive. For Stahl, decomposition was not merely the only reliable *indicator* of death, it was close to being the actual *definition* of death (Dunglison, 1833b; Garrison, 1929b).

Beyond their discoveries in artificial resuscitation, physiologists further complicated the concept of death with series of experiments that raised troubling questions about the relation between the death of an individual and the death of his or her body parts. From antiquity, observers had been perplexed by the survival, for a time, of vital signs in the bodies of decapitated animals and people. The revival of anatomy and experimental vivisection in the seventeenth century confirmed these old findings and the associated concerns as evidence accumulated that the heart, lungs and brain could each function for a considerable time in the absence of the others (Dunglison, 1833a). In fact, the first case of "brain death" to be maintained on a "ventilator" may well have been the decapitated rooster, whose circulation and respiration William Harvey preserved with a bellows in 1627 (Baker, 1971).

The questions now being addressed arose directly from the fact that vital organs could be maintained or terminated separately from each other. At what point in the process, if ever, does the organism as a whole cease to live? At what point does its personal existence end?

Late Nineteenth Century Death

During the late nineteenth century doubts about doctors' ability to define and diagnose death gradually subsided owing in greater part to increasing public faith in medical expertise rather than to new technical innovations. By the end of the century, such issues had almost disappeared as topics of legitimate professional concern. Late nineteenth century physicians demonstrated greatly increased confidence in their ability to recognise death, in part owing to the introduction of precise new technical instruments to test for vital functions (Reiser, 1978). Laennec invented the most important of these tools, the stethoscope, in 1819 and Bouchut was the first to apply this to the systematic diagnosis of death in 1846 (Porter, 1882a; *London Medical Record*, 1874). Electrical tests for neuromuscular function also became more technical and accurate and in 1920 *Scientific American Monthly* labelled the failure to respond to electrical stimulation an "infallible" indicator of death (*Scientific American Monthly*, 1920). Rather than accept any one test as definitive by itself, many physicians combined the best fifteen or twenty such procedures that would adequately ensure that vital functioning had, indeed, ceased. This shotgun approach, originating with Orfila in 1818, became established as professional orthodoxy by the 1880s (Orfila, 1818; Porter, 1882; Capron, 1980).

However, scientific uncertainties continued to result from work in resuscitation, suspended animation and experimental vivisection. Conventional medical wisdom held that previously reported recoveries from apparent death resulted from the insensitivity of earlier diagnostic tools rather than from any actual intermission in the heartbeat and breathing. Late nineteenth century physiological discoveries hardly justified such medical confidence. For example, Schiff, in 1874, used open chest cardiac massage to revive a heart that had stopped beating; this provided dramatic evidence that true cardiac arrest did not mean instant or certain death (Pearson, 1965; Brouardel, 1897; Carrington, 1910). By the 1880s and 1890s, improved resuscitation techniques occasionally produced instances in which lung and heart functions were artificially maintained for many hours, following extensive brain damage. Many, if not most, modern physicians would probably diagnose such cases as "brain dead" and regard them as casting doubt on the value of heart-lung function death tests in some circumstances. However, physicians at the time saw in these patients nothing more than an unusually prolonged confirmation of the ancient doctrine that the heart was the last organ to die (Duckworth, 1898; Pinkus, 1985).

Even as physicians demonstrated their confidence in heart, lung and muscle function tests to diagnose individual death, many physiologists had begun to conclude that individual life depended instead on the nervous system. To the conceptual founder of modern neurophysiology, Sherrington, what distinguished the life of an organism from the lives of its parts was its ability to integrate and co-ordinate those parts, a capability that depended largely on an intact nervous system. For Sherrington, an intact nervous system made possible the integrated functioning that defined a living individual (Sherrington, 1906; Garrison, 1929c; Englehardt, 1975).

Death in the Twentieth Century

Even as the public's fear of premature burial lessened, new advances in medicine and physiology continued to provoke potentially troubling questions about the definition and recognition of death. These findings came in the same fields that had undermined eighteenth century distinctions between life and death, namely resuscitation, suspended animation and the physiological relation between the individual organism and its component parts. In terms of the latter, Carrel between 1910 and 1920 pioneered the culture of cells, tissues and entire organ systems in artificial media outside of the body. Given the proper care, he asserted, our cells were immortal (Middleton, 1914). By the 1940s, Carrel's perfusion techniques made it possible for scientists to maintain separate life in the head and the body of a decapitated dog (Kaempffert, 1953; Newman, 1940). Another application of his techniques allowed the transplantation of organs and the first renal transplant between two living patients came in 1954. As they had since the seventeenth century (Aries, 1981), such organ separations and interchanges seriously complicated the definition of life for a human organism as a whole. For neurologists, however, these organ separation and transplant experiments strongly implicated the brain as being the locus of the integrative activity that constituted individual life (Korein, 1978). With the development of the electroencephalogram (EEG in 1929, neurophysiologists gained the ability to measure a function of the brain directly without relying on other organs as indicators of the brain's vitality. Within a year, Crile had redefined life as the ability to generate spontaneous electric current (Crile, 1930) and by 1941, *Time* magazine reported that the absence of EEG activity was being used as a test for death (*Time*, 1941; Sugar and Gerard, 1938).

If transplantation muddied the concept of individual life, this century's progress in resuscitation made a definition of death even more elusive. Russian scientists, from Bachmetieff in 1910 to Negovskii in the 1960s, produced startling breakthroughs in reviving the seemingly dead, based on their discovery that deep cold enabled animals, including humans, to survive for an hour or more without vital signs (*Review of Reviews*, 1914; Negovskii, 1962). These techniques undoubtedly saved lives in the sense that deaths, that hitherto would have been inevitable, were avoided and life was prolonged for the human being on whom the techniques were practised. However, such techniques also complicated the definition of life and death. The mass media reported such advances but early news accounts of cardiac resuscitation presented it as resurrection (*New York Times*, 1953; *Literary Digest*, 1935; *New York Times*, 1953; Hoehling, 1955); popular articles reported these discoveries under headlines such as "What is death?". Many of these publications admitted that doctors lacked a definitive definition of death and that diagnostic mistakes were still being made (Kaempffert, 1953; Newman, 1940; *Time*, 1941; *Review of Reviews*, 1911).

As early as the 1890s physicians had found occasional brain injury victims whose heart and lung functions could be maintained by continuous artificial ventilation but whose consciousness never returned

(Cushing, 1902; Duckworth, 1898; *Literary Digest*, 1931; Pinkus, 1985). With the spread of improved resuscitation techniques and devices, such cases became common enough for the International Congress of Anaesthesiologists to seek guidance from Pope Pius XII in 1957; his response left it up to the medical profession to clarify the definition of death. Also in the 1950s, the legal system first began to grapple with the problem of distinguishing various types of coma from death. In such early cases as Thomas -v- Anderson (1950) and Smith -v- Smith (1958), both in the USA, the courts initially ruled that a comatose patient remained alive so long as heart and lung vital signs were maintained. However, the development of organ transplantation complicated these issues as early as 1963. The Potter case of that year involved a British physician who had removed a kidney for transplantation from a ventilator-maintained brain damaged donor (Arnold, Zimmerman and Martin, 1968); a similar case was reported in Sweden (Snider, 1967). By the late 1960s, legal definitions of death were in turmoil.

Over the past two decades since the first heart transplants, the medical and legal professions, philosophers and the public have become embroiled in a worldwide debate over redefining death. At first, the ancient fear of premature diagnosis of death and subsequent inappropriate burial was raised (*Newsweek*, 1967), but others such as the advocates of euthanasia began to suggest that the diagnosis of death was too conservative. For the first time, there was both a fear of being wrongly declared dead and a fear of being wrongly declared alive. From the late 1960s to the mid 1970s, most of the efforts to redefine death (including the London Ciba Symposium of 1966 and the 1968 World Medical Association meeting in Sydney) developed as specific responses to organ transplantation. This approach inadvertently convinced both the participants and the public that the issue was unprecedented and arose entirely from new medical technology. In 1968, a Harvard University committee produced the best known of these early attempts at redefinition. This report, written by Beecher, offered a set of criteria for diagnosing "irreversible coma" and emphasised the loss of all brain functions (Beecher, 1968). While the Harvard criteria attempted to measure the end of both conscious and unconscious brain activity, many others took the term "brain death" to mean primarily the permanent loss of consciousness. Brierley *et al*, in 1971, urged that death be defined not as the loss of all brain functions but as the permanent cessation of "those higher functions of the nervous system that demarcate man from the lower primates" (Brierley, Adams, Graham and Simpson, 1971).

The 1981 Presidential Commission report "Defining death", rejected this "higher functions" approach in favour of a "whole brain" definition that emphasised integrative reflexes. The Commission rejected the "higher functions" view because of the lack of agreement on the components of consciousness, because of the lack of reliable tests for it and because the permanent loss of consciousness was compatible with the indefinite continuation of vitality in other organ systems (President's Commission, 1981a). Critics of these findings argue that these problems were merely a reflection of the present limitations of science and medicine and not flaws in the concept of a "higher functions" definition of death (Youngner and Bartlett, 1983). Others have cogently argued that the subjective states of consciousness are inherently inaccessible to others; according to this philosophical tradition, there can never be a method of testing for consciousness because such a test is fundamentally unattainable (Jonas, 1974).

Efforts to formulate "higher brain" definitions of death have continued especially in the academic community, while doubt about the validity of any brain-based definitions of death have also continued, particularly outside the medical profession (Jonas, 1974; Rosner and Bleich, 1979a). While there is no published evidence that death tests for whole-brain functions are any more inaccurate than traditional tests for heart-lung functions (President's Commission, 1981b), highly publicised mistakes seemingly have been made in declaring people brain dead (Arnold, Zimmerman and Martin, 1968b; *Newsweek*, 1967; Roelofs, 1978; Rosner and Bleich, 1979b). Unfortunately, the initial media reports emphasised such errors and the image has remained. In this respect, there are still some troubling gaps in our scientific knowledge about whole-brain death. The President's Commission listed eight not uncommon conditions, ranging from extreme cold to anaesthetic overdose, that are known to depress very significantly the heart rate, breathing and electrical activity of the brain and that are therefore capable of invalidating a determination of death (President's Commission, 1981a). Similar reports have been published by Marshall (1967). The "mistakes" in diagnosing people brain-dead referred to earlier have usually been a result of an incomplete appreciation of these problems. As a result, popular fears of being wrongly declared dead, even using supposedly conservative whole-brain criteria can still claim some justification (Arnold, Zimmerman and Martin, 1968c).

At present, there are four main groups each advocating a different concept of death:

- those who advocate adherence to the traditional beating heart and breathing criteria (Jonas, 1974; Evans, 1990);
- those who advocate a brain-stem concept of death (Pallis, 1983; Lamb, 1985);
- those who advocate whole-brain death (Lynn, 1981);
- those who advocate some form of "higher function" or neocortical brain death (Beecher, 1969; Veatch, 1972; Gervais, 1986; Green and Wickler, 1980).

Defining death is a philosophical activity whilst determining and applying the criteria for declaring that someone is dead are medical activities. Since a definition of death is underpinned by basic beliefs and values, different understandings of death can be held by different people and cultures.

Summary

Both the definition and the diagnosis of death have always been uncertain. Since there never was a "Golden Age of Hearts and Lungs" when defining death was unambiguous and certain, it is irrational to assume that the presently accepted method of diagnosing death in the majority of people, namely lack of beating heart and lack of spontaneous breathing, is more certain at present. However, this does not detract from its role as a standard against which other, different, more specialised methods can be compared.

Death is not simply a timeless and permanently definable term; death has meant different things to different people at different times in history. While the meaning of death in terms of what we believe about death or how we regard death has not changed with time, what has undoubtedly changed, especially in more recent times, is the range of individuals about whom we can all agree that they are all dead. This history of change should lead us to expect future changes any of which may invalidate both the present-day tests and basic definitions.

Finally, this introduction reminds us that untestable definitions of death have tended to be sources of problems both within and without the medical profession. It follows from this that any suggested concept of death should lead to a definition that can be tested rigorously and for which the tests themselves should be as free as possible from influence by other physiological variables.

References

Ackerknecht, E.H. (1968a), "Death in the history of medicine", *Bull. History Medicine*, vol. 42, pp. 19-23.
Ackerknecht, E.H. (1968b), "Death in the history of medicine", *Bull. History Medicine*, vol. 42, p. 21.
Aries, P. (1981), *The hour of our death*, Knopf, New York, pp. 353-361.
Arnold, J.D., Zimmerman, T.F. and Martin D.C. (1968c), "Public attitudes and the diagnosis of death", *J. American Med. Ass.*, vol. 206, pp. 1949-1954.
Arnold, J.D., Zimmerman, T.F. and Martin D.C. (1968a), "Public attitudes and the diagnosis of death", *J. American Med. Ass.*, vol. 206, p. 1950.
Arnold, J.D., Zimmerman, T.F. and Martin D.C. (1968b), "Public attitudes and the diagnosis of death", *J. American Med. Ass.*, vol. 206, p. 1952.
Augustine St. (1972), *The City of God against the pagans*, Loeb Classical Library, Harvard Univ. Press, Cambridge.
Baker, A.B. (1971), "Artificial respiration, the history of an idea", *Medical History*, vol. 15, p. 339.
Beecher, H.K. (1968), "A definition of irreversible coma. Report of the ad hoc committee of the Harvard Medical School to examine the definition of brain death", *Journal American Med. Ass.*, vol. 205, pp. 337-340.
Beecher, H.K. (1969), "After the definition of irreversible coma", *New Eng. J. Medicine*, vol. 281, pp. 1070-1071.
Braid, J. (1850), *Observations on trance; or, human hibernation*, John Churchill, London, p. 57.
Brierley, J.B., Adams, J.H., Graham, D.I. and Simpson, J.A. (1971), "Neocortical death after cardiac arrest", *Lancet*, vol. ii, pp. 560-565.
Brouardel, P.C.H. (1897), *Death and sudden death*, William Wood, New York, pp. 20, 29.
Bynum, W.F., Browne, E.J. and Porter, R. (1981), (eds.), *Dictionary of the History of Science*, Princeton Univ. Press, Princeton, pp. 296-298.
Capron, A.M. (1980a), "'The rigid embrace of the narrow house': premature burial and the signs of death", *Hastings Center Report*, vol. 10, pp. 25-31.
Capron, A.M. (1980b), "'The rigid embrace of the narrow house': premature burial and the signs of death", *Hastings Center Report*, vol. 10, p. 30.
Carrington, H. (1910), "Death: its phenomena", *Annals of Physical Science*, vol. 9, p. 260.
Colhoun, S. (1823), *An essay on suspended animation*, Edward Parker, Philadelphia, pp. 14-15.
Criel, G.W., Telkes, M. and Rowland, A.F. (1930), "The physical nature of death", *Scientific American*, vol. 143, pp. 30-32.
Cullen, W. (1784), *A letter to Lord Cathcart.... concerning the recovery of persons drowned and seemingly dead*, C. Elliott, Edinburgh, p. 4.
Cushing, H. (1902), "Some experimental and clinical observations concerning states of increased intracranial tension", *American Journal of the Medical Sciences*, vol. 124, pp. 377-391.
Darnton, R. (1968), *Mesmerism and the end of the Enlightenment in France*, Harvard Univ. Press, Cambridge, p. 58.
Duckworth, Sir D. (1898), "Some cases of cerebral disease in which the function of respiration entirely ceases for some hours before that of the circulation", *Edinburgh Medical Journal*, vol. 3(2), pp. 145-152.

Dunglison, R. (1833a), *A new dictionary of medical science*, Charles Bowen, Boston, vol. 2, p. 49.
Dunglison, R. (1833b), *A new dictionary of medical science*, Charles Bowen, Boston, vol. 1, p. 576.
Engelhardt, H.T. Jr. (1975), "John Hughlins Jackson and the mind-body relation", *Bulletin of the History of Medicine*, vol. 49, pp. 141-142.
Evans, M. (1990), "A plea for the heart", *Bioethics*, vol. 4(3), pp. 227-231.
Forbes, J. et al. (1845), (eds.), *Cyclopaedia of practical medicine*, Lea & Blanchard, Philadelphia, vol. 1, p. 380.
Garrison, F.H. (1929a), *An introduction to the history of medicine*, 4th ed., W.B. Saunders, Philadelphia, p. 272.
Garrison, F.H. (1929b), *An introduction to the history of medicine*, 4th ed., W.B. Saunders, Philadelphia, p. 312.
Garrison, F.H. (1929c), *An introduction to the history of medicine*, 4th ed., W.B. Saunders, Philadelphia, p. 543.
Gervais, K.G. (1986), *Redefining death*, Yale Univ. Press, New Haven.
Green, M.B. and Wikler, D. (1980), "Brain death and personal identity", *Philosophy and Public Affairs*, vol. 9, pp. 105-133.
Grier, J. (1937), *A history of pharmacy*, Pharmaceutical Press, London, p. 174.
Hawes, W. (1780), *An address to the public on premature death and premature interment*, Author, London, p. 40.
Hoehling, A.A. (1955), "She was dead for 50 minutes", *Reader's Digest*, vol. 66, pp. 49-52.
Jellinek, S. (1947), *Dying, apparent death and resuscitation*, Williams & Wilkins, Baltimore, p. 201.
Jonas, H. (1974), "Against the stream: comments on the definition and re-definition of death", in *Philosophical Eessays: from ancient creed to technological man*, Univ. of Chicago Press, Chicago (reprinted 1980).
Kaempffert, W. (1953), "Physicians are faced with more uncertainty as to the fact of clinical death", *New York Times*, Feb 22, sect. IV: 9, (col. 6).
Kaempffert, W. (1953), "What is clinical death?", *Science Digest*, vol. 34, pp. 76-77.
Kesteven, W.B. (1855), "The signs of death", *British and Foreign Medico-Chirurgical Review*, vol.15, p. 74.
Kite, C. (1788a), *An essay on the recovery of the apparently dead*, C. Dilly, London, p. 101.
Kite, C. (1788b), *An essay on the recovery of the apparently dead*, C Dilly, London, p. 122.
Korein, J. (1978), "*The problem of brain death: development and history*", in J. Korein (ed.), Brain death: interrelated medical and social issues, *Annals of the New York Acad. Sciences*, vol. 315, pp. 19-38.
Lamb, D. (1985), *Death, brain death and ethics*: State Univ. of New York Press, New York.
Lancisi, G.M. (1971a), *De subitaneis mortibus* (On sudden deaths), White, P.D. and Boursy, A.V. (trans.), St John's Univ. Press, New York, p. 42.
Lancisi, G.M. (1971b), *De subitaneis mortibus* (On sudden deaths), White, P.D. and Boursy, A.V. (trans.), St John's Univ. Press, New York, p. 45.
Lee, R.V. (1972), "Cardiopulmonary resuscitation in the eighteenth century", *J. History Medicine and Allied Sciences*, vol. 27, pp. 418-433.
Literary Digest (1931), "Heart-beats after death", *Literary Digest*, vol. 110, p. 28.
Literary Digest (1935), "From beyond the Styx: English gardener tells of experience while heart stopped", *Literary Digest*, vol. 119, Feb. 23, p. 26.
Littel. (1847), "The prevention of premature burials", *Littel's Living Age*, vol. 13, pp. 357-358.

London Medical Record. (1874), "The signs of death. Report on the prizes founded by he Marquis d'Ourches", *London Medical Record*, vol. 2, pp. 205-207, 221-223.

Lynn, J. (1981), "Guidelines for the determination of death. Report of the medical consultants on the diagnosis of death to the President's commission for the study of ethical problems in medicine and biomedical and behavioural research", *J. American Med. Ass.*, vol. 246, pp. 2185-2186.

Marshall, T.K. (1967), "Premature burial", *Medico-legal Journal*, vol. 35, pp. 14-24.

Middleton, J. (1914), "Flesh that is immortal: Dr Alexis Carrel's experiments with tissues of a chicken", *World's Work*, vol. 28, pp. 590-593.

Negovskii, V.A. (1962), *Resuscitation and artificial hypothermia*, Consultants Bureau, New York, esp. p117.

New York Times. (1953), "'Dead', he revives only to die again", *New York Times*, Feb 16, p. 12, col. 6.

New York Times. (1953), "Girl 'dies', then lives 22 hours", *New York Times*, Feb 18, p. 56, col. 3.

Newman, B.M. (1940), "What is death?", *Scientific American*, vol. 162, pp. 336-337.

Newsweek. (1967), "Back from the dead", *Newsweek*, vol. 70, p. 99.

Newsweek. (1967), "When are you really dead?", *Newsweek*, vol. 70, (Dec 18), p. 87.

Orfila, M.J.B. (1818a), *A popular treatise on the remedies to be employed in cases of poisoning and apparent death; including the means.....also of distinguishing real from apparent death*, William Phillips, London, p. 151.

Orfila, M.J.B. (1818b), *A popular treatise on the remedies to be employed in cases of poisoning and apparent death; including the means...also of distinguishing real from apparent death*, William Phillips, London, p. 154.

Pallis, C. (1983), *ABC of brainstem death*, British Medical Assoc., London.

Pearson, J.W. (1965), *Historical and experimental approaches to modern resuscitation*, Charles C. Thomas, Illinois, p. 5.

Pernick, M.S. (1985a), *A calculus of suffering: pain, professionalism and anaesthesia in nineteenth century America*, Columbia Univ. Press, New York, p. 105.

Pernick, M.S. (1985b), *A calculus of suffering: pain, professionalism and anaesthesia in nineteenth century America*, Columbia Univ. Press, New York.

Philip, A.P.W. (1834), "On the nature of death", *Philosophical Transactions of the Royal Society*, vol. 1, pp. 167-198.

Pinkus, R.L. (1985a), "Brain death", *J. Neurosurg.*, vol. 62, pp. 160-161.

Porter, G.L. (1882a), "Recognition of death", *Proceedings of the Connecticut Medical Society*, vol. 2(3), p. 93.

Porter, G.L. (1882b), "Recognition of death", *Proceedings of the Connecticut Medical Society*, vol. 2(3), p. 95.

President's Commission for the study of ethical problems in medicine and biomedical and behavioural research. (1981a), *Defining death: medical, legal and ethical issues in the determination of death*, Government Printing Office, Washington DC.

President's Commission for the study of ethical problems in medicine and biomedical and behavioural research. (1981b), *Defining death: medical, legal and ethical issues in the determination of death*, Government Printing Office, Washington DC, p. 82.

Reaumur, R.A.F. de. (1740), *Avis pour donner du secours a ceux que l'on croit noyes*. Reprinted in Louis, A. (1752), *Lettres sur la certitude des signes de la mort*, Michel Lambert, Paris.

Reiser, S.J. (1978), *Medicine and the reign of technology*, Cambridge Univ. Press, Cambridge.

Review of Reviews. (1911), "What is meant by death?", *Review of Reviews*, vol. 43, pp. 623-624.
Review of Reviews. (1914), "Anabiosis: a state between and betwixt life and death", *Review of Reviews*, vol. 50, pp. 240-242.
Robbins, R.H. (1970), "Signs of death in middle English", *Mediaeval Studies*, vol. 32, pp. 282-298.
Roelofs, R. (1978), "Some preliminary remarks on brain death", in J. Korein (ed.), Brain death: interrelated medical and social issues, *Annals of the New York Acad. Sciences*, vol. 315, p. 42.
Rosner, F. and Bleich, J.D. (1979a), (eds.), *Jewish Bioethics*, Hebrew Publishing Co., Brooklyn, pp. 280-285.
Rosner, F. and Bleich, J.D. (1979a), (eds.), *Jewish Bioethics*, Hebrew Publishing Co., Brooklyn. p. 290.
Rosner, F. and Bleich, J.D. (1979b), (eds.), *Jewish Bioethics*, Hebrew Publishing Co., Brooklyn, p. 299.
Rosner, F. and Bleich, J.D. (1979b), (eds.), *Jewish Bioethics*, Hebrew Publishing Co., Brooklyn, p. 272.
Rosner, F. and Bleich, J.D. (1979c), (eds.), *Jewish Bioethics*, Hebrew Publishing Co., Brooklyn, pp. 297-298.
Rosner, F. and Bleich, J.D. (1979d), (eds.), *Jewish Bioethics*, Hebrew Publishing Co., Brooklyn, pp. 286-305.
Rosner, F. and Bleich, J.D. (1979e), (eds.), *Jewish Bioethics*, Hebrew Publishing Co., Brooklyn, p. 285.
Schechter, D.C. (1971), "Early experience with resuscitation by means of electricity", *Surgery*, vol. 69, pp. 360-372.
Scientific American Monthly (1920), "Fear of being buried alive: infallible signs of death", *Scientific American Monthly*, vol. 1, pp. 396-397.
See, W. (1880), "The extreme rarity of premature burials", *Popular Science Monthly*, vol. 17, p. 529.
Sherrington, C.S. (1906), *The integrative action of the nervous system*, Scribner, New York.
Shrock, N.M. (1835a), "On the signs that distinguish real from apparent death", *Transylvania J. Medicine*, vol. 8, pp. 210-220.
Shrock, N.M. (1835b), "On the signs that distinguish real from apparent death", *Transylvania J. Med.*, vol. 8, pp. 216-218.
Smith, J.G. (1821), *Principles of forensic medicine*, Underwood, London, pp. 28-29.
Smith, J.G. (1827), *Principles of forensic medicine*, Underwood, London, p. 12.
Smith-v-Smith (1958), 229 Ark 579, 317 SW 2d 275.
Snart, J. (1824a), *An historical inquiry concerning apparent death and premature interment*, Sherwood, Neely and Jones, London, p. 81.
Snart, J. (1824b), *An historical inquiry concerning apparent death and premature interment*, Sherwood, Neely and Jones, London, pp. 138-146.
Snider, A. (1967), "When is a person dead?", *Science Digest*, vol. 62, pp. 70-71.
Stevenson, L. (1975a), "Suspended animation", *Bull. History Medicine*, vol. 49, pp. 482-511.
Stevenson, L. (1975b), "Suspended animation", *Bull. History Medicine*, vol. 49, pp. 496-499.
Sugar, O. and Gerard, R.W. (1938), "Anoxia and brain potentials", *J. Neurophysiology*, vol. 1, pp. 558-572.
Symonds, J.A. (1836), "Death", in R.B. Todd (ed.), *Cyclopaedia of anatomy and physiology*, Longman, Brown, Green, Longmans and Roberts, London, p. 791.

Tebb, W. and Vollum, E.P. (1905), in W.R. Hadwen (ed.), *Premature burial and how it may be prevented, with special reference to trance, catalepsy and other forms of suspended animation*, 2nd ed., Swan Sonnenschein, London, p. 219.

Tebb, W. and Vollum, E.P. (1905a), in W.R. Hadwen (ed), *Premature burial and how it may be prevented, with special reference to trance, catalepsy and other forms of suspended animation*, 2nd ed., Swan Sonnenschein, London, p. 409.

Tebb, W. and Vollum, E.P. (1905b), in W.R. Hadwen,(ed), *Premature burial and how it may be prevented, with special reference to trance, catalepsy and other forms of suspended animation*, 2nd ed., Swan Sonnenschein, London, pp. 409-436.

Thomas-v-Anderson. (1950), 96 Cal App 2d 371, 215 P 2d 478.

Time. (1941), "What is death?", *Time*, vol. 37, p. 62.

Veatch, R.M. (1972), "Brain death: welcome definition or dangerous judgement?", *Hastings Center Report*, vol. 2(5), pp. 10-13. (See also Veatch, R.M. "Whole brain, neocortical and higher brain related concepts", in R.M. Zaner (ed.), *Death: beyond whole brain criteria*, Kluwer Academic, Boston, p. 171-186.)

Weiner, P.P. (1968), (ed.), *Dictionary of the History of Ideas*, Scribner, New York, vol. 1, pp. 229-236.

Winslow, J.B. (1740), *An mortis incertae signa minus incerta a chirurgicis, quam ab aliis experimentis?*, Quillau, Paris. (Referred to by Pernick, M.S. (1988), "Back from the grave", in R.M. Zaner (ed.), *Death: beyond whole-brain criteria*, Kluwer Academic Publishers, Dordrecht, p. 21.)

Winslow, J.B. (1746a), *The uncertainty of the signs of death and the danger of precipitate interment*, M. Cooper, London.

Winslow, J.B. (1746b), *The uncertainty of the signs of death and the danger of precipitate interment*, M. Cooper, London, p. 50.

Winslow, J.B. (1746c), *The uncertainty of the signs of death and the danger of precipitate interment*, M. Cooper, London, p. 18.

Youngner, S.J. and Bartlett, E.T. (1983), "Human death and high technology: the failure of the whole brain formulations", *Annals Of Internal Medicine*, vol. 99, pp. 252-258.

2 Current Concepts of Death and Brain Death

"However many ways there may be of being alive, it is certain that there are vastly more ways of being dead"
Richard Dawkins *The Blind Watchmaker*

Introduction

The basic point put forward in the quote at the beginning of this monograph is worth re-iterating here. Dennett's argument is that there is no hope of *discovering* a point at which we can confidently say that death has occurred or that constitutes death—we must *select* a point beyond which we say that death has occurred and provide reasoned argument to support the selection. The development of the concept of brain death illustrates this well.

Whilst I outlined, briefly, in chapter 1 the development of the concept of brain death, some familiarity with the history of application of the brain death concept is likely to be of assistance both in understanding its present status and in anticipating the direction of future developments, and I propose to examine it in greater depth here. The notion of brain death was not, in the first instance, a method to facilitate the identification of patients who would be suitable organ donors for transplantation. The concept of brain death and guidelines for its recognition were developed originally as a means of assisting in making decisions to discontinue treatment in terminally ill or irretrievably ill patients. Traditionally, such decisions were always made for the reason that further treatment could offer no benefit to the patient; the recognition of a state termed "brain death" was intended to supplement by providing another piece of diagnostic information, not to replace, this approach to discontinuation of treatment based upon the interests of the patient. Whilst the definition of the state of brain death occurred independently of the process of identifying potential organ donors, attitudes towards both brain death and the management of patients diagnosed as brain dead have been influenced by advances in transplant surgery.

Recognition of Brain Death

The first successful cardiac transplant on 3 December 1967 changed dramatically the climate that had prevailed until then, namely that an individual was alive until the last cardiac contraction. This change was, effectively, to separate cessation of cardiac function from death. The operation performed in December 1967 demonstrated that life need not cease with the cessation of an individual's heart, but that cardiac function and life could thereafter be regarded as separable entities.

There were, however, difficulties with brain death as Toole (1971) pointed out

> "unlike the traditional moment of death, upon which layman and physician have always agreed, the end point chosen for certification of brain death is a matter of opinion not obvious to everyone".

This opinion from Toole does overstate the case, however, inasmuch as the traditional moment of death upon which both layman and physician have agreed has not always been the moment of death and the agreement has not always existed (see chapter 1). In addition, the formal definition of brain death varies in different geographical areas. The earliest of the statements on brain death, the report of the *ad hoc* committee of the Harvard Medical School (Beecher, 1968a), seems to have examined the problem of brain death with a preconceived idea of the end result, in view of the opening sentence of the report—"Our primary purpose is to define irreversible coma as a new criterion for death". The "Harvard criteria" established in 1968 by this report have shaped subsequent attitudes in regard to brain death in both the United States of America and, to a lesser extent, Britain. A major influence of the Harvard committee report has been the establishment, in the USA, of the requirement for evidence of cessation of function of the whole brain and the more recent authoritative statement on brain death by the President's Commission for the study of ethical problems in medicine and biomedical and behavioural research (Lynn, 1981) affirmed that "an individual with irreversible cessation of all functions of the entire brain, including the brainstem, is dead". In contrast to this concept of brain death being the irretrievable loss of function of the whole brain, the British definition of brain death is based exclusively upon the irretrievable loss of function of the brainstem. The conference of the Medical Royal Colleges stated in 1976 that "It is agreed that permanent functional death of the brainstem constitutes brain death" (Conference,

1976). The criteria for death enumerated in the report were considered to be "sufficient to distinguish between those patients who retain the functional capacity to have a chance of even partial recovery and those in whom no such possibility exists". In effect, the report was saying that its specification of the brainstem, rather than the whole brain, was based on the predictive value of its permanent loss of function rather than on any proposition that the brain stem was, functionally, a central and indispensable part of the whole brain. However, a second report from the conference in 1979 changes that and took the position that "brain death represents the stage at which a patient becomes truly dead, because by then all functions of the brain have permanently and irreversibly ceased" (Conference, 1979). Comparison of the statements in 1976 and 1979 lead to the conclusion that the 1979 statement upgraded the interpretation of the clinical criteria recommended in 1976 from being predictive of death to being death itself. In other words, in 1976 brainstem death was thought to be merely prognostic of human death, that is brainstem death was equivalent to brain death and brain death was associated with a uniformly fatal prognosis. However, in 1979, the position had changed to that of brainstem death being equivalent to brain death and that brain death was death itself and not a mere predictor of death. In a discussion of the differences between brain death as defined in the USA and Britain, and simultaneously noting that Canada differs from both countries in its requirements for brain death, a report stated that "clinical criteria make it possible to be brain dead in one country and not in another" (Levin and Whyte, 1988). This is an unsatisfactory state of affairs and some close examination of the reasons for the selection of the brain as the important organ in the determination of death is indicated.

Basis for the Selection of the Brain as the Important Organ in the Determination of Death

As I have indicated in the previous section, the idea of brain death arose in response to the recognition that there was a group of patients with irreversible brain damage of such an extent that suspension of artificial ventilation would result in permanent cessation of respiration and, consequently, of cardiac contraction. The cessation of function of the heart and lungs was traditionally accepted as indicative of death. The criteria for brain death emerged as a result of retrospective analysis of the clinical features of brain injured patients whose subsequent clinical course

provided confirmatory evidence that irreversible loss of brain function had occurred. Much has been written about the requirements for the diagnosis of "death of the brain", and with regard to the question of why the brain was selected as the organ the failure of which should be identified with death. A list of possible reasons, although not exhaustive, would include:
- following irreversible cessation of brain function, all other organ systems will inevitably cease to function;
- unlike other organ systems, brain function, once lost, is irreplaceable;
- irreversible loss of brain function entails permanent loss of consciousness;
- irreversible loss of brain function entails permanent loss of sentience;
- irreversible loss of brain function entails permanent loss of the integrative function of the brain;
- recognition of death on the basis of loss of brain function is doing no more than recognising overtly the reason underlying the traditional diagnosis of death following cessation of the blood circulation (McCullagh, 1993a).

Whilst I discuss my reservation about the present concepts of brain death later, in chapter 4, it is pertinent to examine these suggestions at this point since they are not all dealt with later. McCullagh (1993b) deals with these points in a robust fashion and I shall borrow from him. Equating the irreversible loss of brain function with death is based on the belief that cessation of function of all other organ systems will inevitably follow brain death, irrespective of maintenance of "life support" systems. While this belief appears to be true, and the inevitability of the cessation of function of the other organ systems after cessation of brain function is undoubted, this equating of brain death with death is essentially a substitution of a forecast of a future clinical state for the present clinical state. As McCullagh (1993c) argues, "unless one is prepared consistently to adopt the position that a hopeless outlook justifies the presumption that the outlook has already been fulfilled, this argument would seem to have substantial limitations".

The irreplaceability of the brain and hence of brain functions has been advanced as a reason for regarding brain death and death as identical. Whilst the technology to replace other organ systems, notably heart, lung, liver and kidney, either by organ transplantation or by prosthetic devices has been advancing, there is no comparable substitution of brain function (at least of the higher brain functions) at present or in prospect. However, Jonas discussed the possibility of substitution of brainstem functions by some external device and argued that the resultant patient would not be considered dead because of the non-spontaneity of the brainstem function in the same way that a patient with a transplanted heart or a totally artificial heart would not be considered dead (Jonas, 1974a). This suggestion by Jonas, made in 1970, is not, perhaps, as unlikely as it may seem at first sight. Ventilation can be maintained in an individual with a high cervical cord transection (which has resulted in paralysis of breathing) by stimulating the nerves that normally carry the impulses needed for spontaneous respiration by means of an implanted nerve stimulator; the patient so treated appears to be breathing spontaneously. There is no technological reason why this technique could not be used in patients in whom the loss of spontaneous respiration was a result of brainstem dysfunction. The basic question is whether the irreversible loss of spontaneity of function is adequate for a diagnosis of death when the loss involves the brain but not when it involves the heart or, indeed, any other organ that can be transplanted at the present time.

The irreversible loss of consciousness that occurs with brain death has been claimed by some as a reason for equating brain death with death. Some claim that it is the actual irreversible loss of consciousness that is important (Beecher, 1968b) while others argue that some other feature which is dependent upon the presence of consciousness is the important feature (Gervais, 1986; Veatch, 1975; Cranford and Smith, 1988); I will classify them together for this discussion although I deal with them separately elsewhere (chapters 3 and 4). In all cases, the clinical state of permanent unconsciousness, or the persistent vegetative state (PVS), is proposed as death. A major objection to the view that permanent unconsciousness is an infallible indicator of cessation of brain function, let alone death, could be that such an argument fails to allow for the possibility of subconscious activity in such a brain damaged individual (McCullagh, 1993d). McCullagh discusses this at some length and argues that consciousness has acquired much of its importance because of its prerequisite rôle for expression of the human potential for rationality and suggests that a valid case could be argued that subconscious activity is also likely to be an exclusive feature of human beings. If this were accepted, then in permanent unconsciousness there would remain an exclusive feature of human beings. This would be an argument against those who advocate adopting the permanent loss of consciousness as the sole criterion for death (Beecher, 1968b, Gervais, 1986; Veatch, 1975; Cranford and Smith, 1988). The loss of sentience, in particular the loss of any capacity to appreciate pain, has been advanced as a reason for accepting brain death as death. This line of reasoning is applied especially to anencephalic infants and to the foetus. However, the loss of sentience in an individual according to Jonas (1974b) merely demonstrates that the individual concerned has crossed the boundary between being sentient and no longer being sentient, not the boundary between life and death. (I shall return to this form of argument later in chapter 8.)

Loss of the integrative function of the brain, consequent upon brain death, has been put forward as a reason for equating brain death with death by Lamb (1985). He concedes that organs other than the brain (such as liver, heart or skin) are necessary for life and that this apparent arbitrariness in selecting the brain as the prime organ of importance in the determination of death is not merely due to its irreplaceability (a point I have commented on earlier in this chapter) but is due to its rôle as a supreme regulator and co-ordinator. This suggested reason for equating brain death with death is the one that I wish to argue later in this monograph but I will advance my own, independent arguments for its adoption.

The last of the reasons in the list, that is that brain death is no more than a representation of the conventional concept of death is one that I address in chapter 10 and again in chapter 11. McCullagh's response to this argument that brain death is merely one form of the more conventional concept of death is to argue that it is unlikely that physicians in the "pre-brain death" era actually considered that death occurred when there was permanent cessation of heart beat, and that that death occurred as a result of the consequences of the cessation of heart beat for the function of the brain (McCullagh, 1993e). It is much more likely that physicians in the "pre-brain era" considered that death had occurred when there was permanent cessation of heartbeat and breathing simply because these two events had occurred. In this matter of what physicians in the "pre-brain death" era thought was happening when death occurred, I am inclined to agree with McCullagh that the physicians at that time were concerned only with the cessation of heartbeat and breathing and not with any other physiological explanation involving the brain. However, McCullagh's general position on brain death, that is that brain death is a predictor of human death and not death itself, is one that I cannot share. I believe that brain death is death itself and I will put forward arguments for my position in this monograph.

Variation in Brain Death Criteria and Present Position

The existence of geographically determined variations in protocols for the diagnosis of brain death has already been mentioned. One obvious example of this variability is in the criteria for apnoea. The basis of the tests for apnoea (lack of breathing) is to raise the level of carbon dioxide in the blood to a level that is sufficient to stimulate the respiratory centre in an intact brain to respond and initiate breathing. There is some variability in the numerical value of the level of carbon dioxide used in this test and this has led to the observations that "no single standardised method of apnoea testing has gained wide acceptance" (Belsh, Blatt and Schiffman, 1986) and that an individual could be declared legally dead in one jurisdiction and not in another (Levin and Whyte, 1988), a fact that I have already alluded to earlier in this chapter. A quite different criticism of the choice of hypercarbia as the test for apnoea has been made by Evans (personal communication) who has suggested that it is only the need for transplant organs that requires this focus on the hypercarbic drive for respiration and that anoxia is the ultimate respiratory drive. While it is true that anoxia could be considered to be the ultimate respiratory drive, it is also true that the normal respiratory drive, that is the respiratory drive used normally by normal human beings, is hypercarbia (or, more accurately, the partial pressure of carbon dioxide in the blood); anoxia would drive respiration but the high levels of carbon dioxide (hypercarbia) that would inevitably accompany the anoxia would provide a much more powerful respiratory drive. With regard to the testing for brain death, anoxia could never be used as a test for the loss of respiratory drive since the anoxia itself would cause irreversible neurological injury. Hypercarbia is used because it is a more powerful physiological drive for respiration and normal levels of oxygen in the blood can be maintained during the test, thereby ensuring that no further damage (as a result of hypoxia or anoxia) is inflicted. This explains why hypercarbia (in preference to anoxia or hypoxia) is used as a test for the respiratory drive in brainstem and brain death testing. This argument in rebuttal of Evans' suggestion presupposes that brain death is an acceptable concept and for Evans (1990) it is not; however, it remains the case that hypercarbia is used for sound physiological reasons, namely that it is the normal and most powerful drive to breathing.

Whilst the original concepts of brain death envisaged the loss of all brain function or total brain death, these concepts have changed with time. Sweet (1978) argued that "it makes no practical difference if some hundreds of thousands of the many millions of brain cells are still functional, and it is certainly impractical at present to test the function of all brain cell clusters". This change reflects, I think, the essentially practical nature of medicine and the development of a pragmatic solution to a problem, which is that we cannot know whether or not all brain cells are dead in an individual who has been diagnosed as "brain dead". However, it does represent a significant change from the original concept, and in the same article the question was raised "What percentage of brain cells could remain alive without altering the patient's status from that of being brain dead?". The acceptance of brain death as a state that is not inconsistent with the retention of some detectable brain function has been adopted by a variety of groups both inside (Wetzel, Setzer, Stiff and Rogers, 1985) and outside medicine (Beecher, 1968b, Gervais, 1986; Veatch, 1975; Cranford and Smith, 1988). However, it is doubtful if the concepts of death and brain death in the community reflect these changes. Comments in the press about multiple "deaths" of the same individual do not help (Frame, 1995), nor does the statement from a judge in Florida that "this lady is dead and has been dead and she is kept alive artificially" (*New York Times*, 1976).

At present, there are two versions of the brain death concept of death that are in common usage, by which I mean that they are accepted by official medical and legal bodies:
- Brainstem death. This has been adequately described by Pallis (Pallis, 1983; Pallis, 1985) and defined by the Royal Colleges (Conference, 1976; Conference 1979).
- Whole brain death. This has been defined by the President's Commission (Lynn, 1981).

However, other concepts of death have been put forward which may be adopted in the future and since I will be discussing these throughout the monograph, it would be useful to introduce them here. These other concepts of death are all based upon the loss of all or some of the higher functions of the brain, that is the functions that depend upon the presence of consciousness; all the advocates of these concepts argue that death has occurred while an individual still breathes spontaneously and, indeed, is able to maintain bodily integrity. This is a significant difference from both the traditional concept of death and the original notion of brain death. I shall consider later (chapter 3) the clinical conditions that could give rise to an individual with such features, but it is appropriate that we examine, at this stage, the claims of the other suggested concepts of death.

Calls for the adoption of a change in the definition of brain death began not long after the introduction of the original idea. A report of the

British Transplantation Society, in 1975, stated that it "saw no objection to the diagnosis of death based on irreversible cessation of cerebral function provided the great majority of ordinary people were aware, and accepted, that doctors were using the word 'death' in this way" (Zaner, 1988). In the USA, the case of Karen Quinlan raised the level of debate both inside and outside the medical profession about the differences between brain death and cerebral death (that is the permanent cessation of function of the cerebral hemispheres) (Beresford, 1978), although some semantic confusion existed as Korein (1978) pointed out. The arguments that have been developed in an attempt to establish cerebral death as the death of a human being have centred, recently, upon the proposition that cerebral death is equal to cessation of existence as a person. Green and Wickler's paper, in 1980, is a good example of this with the argument that brain death (and hence death) has occurred when individual identity has been lost; the authors equated the loss of cerebral function with loss of personal identity (Green and Wickler, 1980). A similar position is taken by Cranford and Smith (1988) and Gervais (1986) inasmuch as they argue that consciousness is the most important standard for human personhood and that personhood is lost in cerebral death. Other criteria, even less well defined have been proposed. Veatch, who has written extensively on this topic, advocates that "our concept of death must be further refined, and our technical criteria for death must be modified accordingly, so that our concept and criteria most accurately reflect our understanding of what is essentially significant to the nature of man" (Veatch, 1975; Veatch 1989). Our concept of death and the criteria for death must indeed be more refined if we are to use a criterion like "what is essentially significant to the nature of man" since I suspect that such a phrase would engender vigorous and prolonged debate about its meaning (not to mention how it would be measured). The concept of death put forward by Bartlett and Youngner, that is the irreversible loss of cognition (Bartlett and Youngner, 1988), seems to be a less nebulous one but like that proposed by Veatch (1975, 1989) is concerned only with functions that appear to be confined to the human species; I shall return to this point in chapter 4.

In essence, what has happened is that the original concept of brain death has been changed from "whole brain death" via "brainstem death" to "cerebral death" and we are now being asked to consider a concept of death that would allow an individual to be diagnosed as "dead" and yet still breathe spontaneously and maintain most, if not all, vital bodily functions.

Current Concepts of Brain Death

There are a variety of brain-centred concepts of death advocated at present, some accepted by legal or government bodies as being sufficient for their respective purposes and others that are not so accepted by official bodies but which continue to be advocated and discussed within philosophical circles. These latter concepts have been described as the "next step forward" in the evolution of the concept of death by Pucetti (1988). All of the brain-centred concepts of death can be classified by the area of brain whose function is required to be permanently lost in order that the criteria for death be satisfied, namely whole brain death, brainstem death and neocortical death. I intend to discuss these concepts of death under this classification.

Whole Brain Death

The first published concept of death that was brain-centred was that of the Harvard Medical School's Ad Hoc Committee, chaired by Beecher, in 1968 (Beecher, 1968a). This advocated simple criteria:
- unreceptivity and unresponsitivity to externally applied stimuli and "inner need";
- absence of spontaneous muscular movements or spontaneous respiration;
- no elicitable reflexes;
- a "flat" or isoelectric EEG (electroencephalogram) (the report stated that this criterion was not essential but was of "great confirmatory value").

These criteria assess not only higher brain functions but also brainstem and spinal cord activity. In 1971, the University of Minnesota Health Sciences Center published the "Minnesota criteria" (Cranford, 1978). These differed from the Harvard criteria in not requiring an EEG and not requiring the absence of movement in response to a painful stimulus. In 1981, the President's Commission (Lynn, 1981) proposed a set of criteria including the standard condition of deep coma and absence of brainstem reflexes including apnoea. The Commission required that the clinical indicators for the cessation of all brain functions must be present for at least 6 hours and confirmation of the clinical findings by EEG was desirable. Further testing for the absence of cerebral blood flow (CBF) could aid in the diagnosis. This latter standard (that is, the one proposed by the President's

Commission) is now the commonly accepted standard for brain death in the USA.

The criteria described above all demand whole brain death as the only clinical state that will satisfy the criteria proposed. However, the clinical state of whole brain death is also demanded by Walton (1983) although he does not advocate criteria that would necessarily need whole brain death in order to be satisfied. His criterion for death is the permanent loss of consciousness and this could be satisfied by neocortical death (that is, the death of the neocortex of the brain (see later section) and also by brainstem death (see later section) but Walton, like others who advocate the permanent loss of consciousness as a criterion for death, takes some pains to argue that it is the permanent loss of consciousness and only the permanent loss of consciousness that matters in the determination of the status of a human being in terms of being alive or dead. Walton's argument for demanding whole brain death in preference to neocortical death (which is demanded by others who advocate the permanent loss of consciousness) is that whole brain death is the safer option. He argues that in the diagnosis of death, while the possibility of treating a dead human being as alive is to be avoided, the possibility of treating a live human being as dead is totally unacceptable and that it is only possible to avoid doing so if whole brain death is adopted as a criterion for death (assuming, of course, that Walton's concept of death is to be adopted in the first place).

Brainstem Death

There are two main advocates of brainstem death as a criterion for death, although each approaches the concept of death differently. The concept of death proposed by Pallis (1983, 1985) is that death has occurred when a human being has permanently lost consciousness and ceased to breathe. He argues strongly for this concept in his monograph (Pallis, 1983) and his arguments have played a major rôle in establishing brainstem death not only as an acceptable form of death but also as the legally accepted form of brain death in the UK. The tests derived from this concept of death and its criteria are all tests of brainstem function, although not all brainstem functions are tested—a fact that I will explore and discuss later in this section.

Lamb (1985) also supports brainstem death but arrives at this point by arguing for a concept of death that consists of the permanent loss of the integrative function of a human being. He places this integrative function in the brainstem and, if this argument were accepted, then logically brainstem death would lead to permanent loss of this function. This is an attempt to present a human being as an integrated, whole organism and not, as Pallis seems to do, as a collection of functions. While I would agree with the concept of death as the permanent loss of the integrative functions of a human being (although I would not necessarily restrict myself to human beings as Lamb and Pallis have), I would disagree with the locus of death advocated by Lamb, that is the brainstem. My own concept of death is elaborated upon later in this monograph.

I must now return to the point that I made earlier in this section that in testing for brainstem death, not all functions of the brainstem are tested. There have been a number of papers describing empirical data that suggest that not all brainstem functions are lost at a time when brainstem death could be diagnosed under the present UK criteria. In addition, there have also been papers suggesting that significant other areas of the brain are not dead—their function has not been lost—at the time of the diagnosis of brainstem death. There is empirical evidence that oesophageal muscle activity (Aitkenhead and Thomas, 1987; Sinclair, 1987; Hill, 1987) and haemodynamic responses occur (Wetzel, Setzer, Stiff and Rogers, 1985); both of these functions depend critically upon the functioning of part of the brainstem. It would seem, therefore, that at the time when the diagnosis of brainstem death could be made under the present criteria in the UK, not all the brainstem is dead. There is also evidence that the pituitary gland continues to function at a time when the diagnosis of brainstem death is possible under the present UK criteria (Fackler and Rogers, 1987; Hall, Mashiter, Lumley and Robson, 1980; Schrader, Krogness, Aakvaag, Sortland and Pusvis, 1980; Robertson, Hramiak and Gelb, 1989). This indicates that brainstem death does not necessarily entail or imply death of other parts of the brain. From this data it is possible to conclude that the control of homeostasis could persist for some time after the diagnosis of brainstem death could be reached if ventilation of the patient continues. In fairness and to balance the argument, it should also be stated that eventually all oesophageal muscle activity, haemodynamic responses and hypothalamic-pituitary function ceases at some time after brainstem death. In short, brainstem death as presently formulated in the UK does not mean death of the whole brainstem nor loss of all brainstem function; nor does it mean, at the time of diagnosis, death of all other areas of the brain outside the brainstem.

Neocortical Death

There are a variety of advocates for neocortical death to be adopted as death of a person; the group of advocates is not, however, homogeneous and there are a variety of concepts of death that are put forward and that could be satisfied by the clinical condition of neocortical death or persistent vegetative state (PVS) as described by Brierley and Graham (1971) in pathological terms and by Jennett and Plum in clinical terms (1972). Beecher (1968a), Cranford and Smith (1988) and Gervais (1986) independently argue for consciousness being the important feature that should be used in the determination of death of a person, Green and Wickler suggest that it is psychological continuity (Green and Wickler, 1980), Pucetti argues for the capacity for personal experience (Pucetti, 1988) and Veatch is of the opinion that the capacity for social interaction is the all-important feature that should be used to determine a person's status in respect of being alive or dead (Veatch, 1975; Veatch, 1989).

Operational Significance of Brain-centred Concepts of Death

So far in this chapter I have put forward a short statement about the history of the development of the concept of brain death and how this concept has changed and been misunderstood. I have, in addition, summarised the present forms of brain death that are commonly discussed and debated, notably brainstem death, whole brain death and neocortical death. I would now like to discuss the significance of the adoption of a brain-centred concept of death upon the practical procedures related to the diagnosis of death.

In the history of the diagnosis of death in medicine, there have been many changes in both the criteria and the tests for death and a summary of these changes was discussed in chapter 1. One common thread running through all these changes, however, was the constant, unchanging concept of death. This concept was the one provided (at least in the Western Hemisphere) by the prevailing religious belief that death occurred when the soul departed from the body. I will discuss later the lack of logical connection between this concept of death and the criteria and tests for death associated with it (see chapter 4); Veatch has provided a thorough analysis of this inconsistency (Veatch 1989). The introduction of brain-centred concepts of death is a significant departure from the older concept of death both intellectually and in terms of criteria and tests for

death. Not surprisingly, therefore, there are operational changes as a result of the introduction of brain-centred concepts of death. These changes can be summarised as follows:
- changes in the identification of the physiological system deemed important for the determination of death and taken as the locus of the tests for death;
- changes to the tests for death (a change that follows from above) and to the complexity of the tests for death;
- changes to the necessary location of the patient at the time that tests for death are performed;
- changes to the qualifications needed by the qualified person who would perform the tests;
- duplication or repetition of the tests by more than one medical practitioner.

I would now like to expand on this summary of the operational changes and indicate the significance of each in turn.

Changes in the Identification of the Physiological System Deemed Important for the Determination of Death and Taken as the Locus for the Tests for Death

Of all the operational changes that necessarily occur as a result of the adoption of a brain-centred concept of death, this change is the most obvious. The change consists of adopting the brain as the organ to be considered the important organ in terms of determination of death in place of the traditional reliance on the heart and breathing. The criteria developed from brain-centred concepts of death and the traditional concepts of death (accepting, for the moment, that the traditional criteria can be derived from the traditional concept) do not show any overlap and the appropriate tests for each of the criteria, again, do not have any overlap. In other words, there is nothing in common between the traditional concept of death and its criteria and tests and the brain-centred concepts of death and their appropriately derived criteria and tests for death. This is the most significant change of all the changes consequent upon the adoption of a brain-centred concept of death and all the other operational changes arise from this alteration. This change in the physiological system that is considered the important system for the determination of death is independent of the precise version of a brain-centred concept of death that is adopted. It is of no matter, in terms of the change to the physiological system chosen for criteria and tests, whether one adopts brainstem death, neocortical death, whole brain death or hypothalamic death (as I advocate in this monograph)—the operational change, that is from using the heart and breathing to using the brain as the system to be examined, is the same. (I have detailed later (see chapter 11) the criteria for my proposed concept of death and the associated tests.) Others may argue that this assertion that the precise version of brain-centred concept of death does not make a difference to the physiological system considered important for the determination of death is not accurate. It could be argued that brainstem death can be diagnosed by reference to physiological systems moderated by the brainstem but neocortical death could not be diagnosed by reference to the same systems; the diagnosis of neocortical death would require reference to the physiological systems moderated by the neocortex, for instance, social interaction (to use Veatch's criterion (1989)). While this argument may have some merit, I suspect that the crux of the matter is how one defines the brain and the various different functional areas within it. If the brain is accepted as a system, then the various different functional areas within it can either be defined as systems in their own right, thereby making the argument about the different versions of a brain-centred concept of death being based on different systems a valid one; or the various different functional areas within the brain could be defined as sub-systems of the brain and in this latter case, my original assertion that the precise choice of version of brain-centred concept of death makes no difference to the physiological system chosen is a valid assertion. In either case, I do not think that my assertion that the change from the cardiovascular and respiratory systems to the central nervous system as the system of importance in the determination of death is an important operational change occurring as a direct result of the adoption of a brain-centred concept of death, can be seriously questioned.

Changes to the Tests for Death and to the Complexity of the Tests for Death

The changes to the tests themselves are consequent upon the changes to the concept of death and to the criteria for death that have resulted from the change of physiological system that is considered important for the determination of death. The traditional tests of listening for a heartbeat and breathing are no longer appropriate under a brain-centred concept of death and tests of a variety of functions of the brain have been put in their place; the exact tests to be performed in the brain-centred concepts of death depend upon the precise concept that is adopted. In the UK, the tests are tests of brainstem function and in the case of my proposed concept of death, the tests are in chapter 11. In all concepts of brain death, there are more than two tests to be performed and the adoption of a brain-centred concept of death would, therefore, result in an increase in the number of tests to be performed, since under the traditional concept, criteria and tests for death there are only two tests, namely tests for cessation of breathing and heartbeat.

However, not only would there be an increase in the number of tests to be performed if a brain-centred concept of death were adopted, there would also be an increase in the complexity of the tests. The traditional tests for death under the traditional concept of death, namely listening with a stethoscope for breath sounds and hearts sounds, are simple procedures taught to all medical students at an early stage in training and have been part of the standard medical investigations for several generations. The tests for death derived from brain-centred concepts of death are not so straightforward. If I restrict myself to the standard brain-centred concept of death in the UK, namely brainstem death, the tests consist of detailed examinations of the cranial nerves arising from the brainstem; this is much more complex, is not in the general armamentarium of medical practitioners and requires specialist training. These tests consist of:

- coma with apnoea;
- absence of brainstem reflexes:
  1. no pupillary response to light;
  2. no corneal reflex;
  3. no vestibulo-ocular reflex;
  4. no gag or reflex responses to tracheal suction.

I shall discuss a consequence of this increase in the complexity of the tests later (see later section in this chapter).

Changes to the Necessary Geographical Position of the Patient at the Time that Tests for Death are Performed

Under the older, widely-used criteria of death (permanent cessation of the beating heart and spontaneous breathing), the tests for death could be applied in any geographical site and did not require that the patient be in any special place prior to the performance of the tests—for example the patient could be at home, outside or in hospital. Under most proposed brain-centred concepts of death, including my own, this wide range of acceptable geographical sites in which the appropriate tests for death may be performed is no longer possible. If I leave to one side for the moment the clinical state of persistent vegetative state which has been suggested by Beecher (1970), Gervais (1986) and others (Green and Wickler, 1980; Bartlett and Youngner, 1988; Veatch, 1989) to be death and restrict my comments to the brain-centred concepts of death that are in use at present, it is a matter of fact that the tests for death under these concepts are all performed in all cases in specialised areas within hospitals, namely intensive care (or therapy) units (ICU or ITU). This is obviously a significant departure from previous practice under the older, traditional criteria and tests for death. It could be argued that both this change of location and restriction of location are requirements of the criteria and tests of the brain-centred concepts of death inasmuch as all patients undergoing these tests are required to be apnoeic and as a result of this apnoea, location in an ICU or ITU is a matter of necessity in order that artificial ventilation be given to the patient. Equally, it could be argued that this restriction of location is not a requirement of the criteria of brain-centred concepts of death but that it is a direct requirement or result of the clinical condition of the patient; in other words, the patient required ventilation or intensive treatment and only after admission to the ITU or ICU and some clinical deterioration did it appear that the patient was brain dead. I would suggest that the restriction of location for the performance of the tests for death under brain-centred concepts of death is a contingent and not a necessary operational change occasioned by the adoption of a brain-centred concept of death.

I would now like to return to the clinical condition of the persistent vegetative state, briefly mentioned in the paragraph above. This clinical condition which is described in detail in chapter 3, does not require artificial ventilation and, therefore, a patient in this condition would not be required to be in an ICU or ITU or even in hospital. It follows from this that the tests for death in this state (if one adopts the arguments that this clinical state should be adopted as death, which I do not accept) could be performed in as wide a range of geographical locations as could the tests for death under the older criteria. Therefore, for this particular state there would be no necessary operational change in respect of the range of geographical sites in which the tests for death could be performed, assuming, of course, that this particular clinical state was formally adopted as death.

Changes to the Qualifications Needed by the Qualified Person who would Perform the Tests

Under the traditional criteria and tests for death, all medical practitioners are able to diagnose death using the appropriate tests and this ability is recognised by the legal system in the UK and other countries. However, this general ability and legal sanction given to all medical practitioners to diagnose death was altered when the brainstem death concept of death and the derived criteria and tests were adopted in the UK. Under present UK guidelines the person checking that the criteria have been complied with and performing the tests must be qualified for 5 years and experienced in the performance of the tests for death. (Experience in the performance of the tests can be obtained in the neurological examination of live patients in which, of course, the results of the tests are quite different from those obtained from the brainstem dead patient.) This demand for familiarity with the tests is a direct result of the increased complexity of the tests that, in the case of brainstem death in the UK, test the function of the cranial nerves that arise within the brainstem. These two changes to the qualifications of the medical practitioner performing the tests have the obvious result that not all medical practitioners are qualified to perform brainstem death tests; this is an obvious and significant operational change that is a direct result of the introduction of a brain-centred concept of death.

Duplication or Repetition of the Tests by More Than One Medical Practitioner

Under the traditional criteria and tests for death, only one medical practitioner was (and still is) required to diagnose death; no second opinion is required. While it is true that two medical practitioners are required to sign a cremation certificate, this certificate does not certify death and the death certificate itself is only required to be signed by one medical practitioner. This set of circumstances is not the case within the UK in relation to brainstem death. If a patient is to be declared dead using brainstem death criteria and tests, then the tests must be performed separately by two appropriately qualified medical practitioners (see above for what is meant by "appropriately qualified"). This is the only circumstance in the UK in which a second medical practitioner must confirm the diagnosis of death. Again, this is a major operational change that has arisen as direct result of the adoption of a brain-centred concept of death.

From this discussion of the operational changes that would occur with the adoption of a brain-centred concept of death, one could put forward the hypomonograph that the diagnosis of death is more secure under the adopted concept of death since two more experienced and more qualified medical practitioners must agree on the diagnosis after independent performance of the tests for death under more controlled conditions than is usual with the more traditional criteria and tests. While this may be the case, and I am not arguing for or against this hypomonograph at present, there are no empirical data to suggest that the diagnosis of death under the more traditional criteria and tests is not secure.

Summary

In this chapter I have put forward a short statement about the history of the development of the concept of brain death and how this concept has changed and been misunderstood. I have, in addition, summarised the present forms of brain death that are commonly discussed and debated, namely brainstem death, whole brain death and neocortical death. I have also indicated that, as a result of the adoption of a brain-centred concept of death (brainstem death) in the UK, the operational changes that have occurred are the physiological system to be examined for the tests for death (has been changed from two to one) but the number of tests to be performed, and the complexity of the tests, has been increased. In addition, death can only be diagnosed in a specific site in a hospital and requires two more qualified and more experienced medical practitioners to make the diagnosis in contrast to the single medical practitioner required under the traditional criteria and tests. These alterations in the way in which death is diagnosed constitute a significant change and are a direct result of the adoption of a brain-centred concept of death.

References

Aitkenhead, A.R. and Thomas D.I. (1987), "Lower oesophageal activity as an indicator of brain death in paralysed and mechanically ventilated patients with head injury", *Brit. Med. J.*, vol. 294, p. 1287.

Bartlett, E.T. and Youngner, S.J. (1988), "Human death and the destruction of the neocortex", in R.M. Zaner (ed.), *Death: beyond whole brain criteria*, Kluwer Academic Publishers, Boston, pp. 199-216.

Beecher, H.K. (1968a), "A definition of irreversible coma. Report of the ad hoc committee of the Harvard Medical School to examine the definition of brain death", *J. American Med. Ass.*, vol. 205, pp. 337-340.

Beecher, H.K. (1970), "The new definition of death, some opposing views", Unpublished paper presented at the American Association for the Advancement of Science, Dec. 1970. (Quoted Tomlinson, T. (1984), "The conservative use of the brain death criteria: a critique", *J. Med. and Philosophy*, vol. 9(4), pp. 377-393 and by Veatch, R.M. (1975), "The whole brain oriented concept of death: an outmoded philosophical formulation", *J. Thanatology*, vol. 3, pp. 13-30.) See also Beecher, H.K. (1969), "After the 'definition of irreversible coma'", *New Eng. J. Med.*, vol. 281, p. 1070.

Beecher, H.K. (1968b), "A definition of irreversible coma", *J. American Med. Ass.*, vol. 205, pp. 337-340.

Belsh, J.M., Blatt, R. and Schiffman, P.L. (1986), "Apnoea testing in brain death", *Arch. Internal Med.*, vol. 146, pp. 2385-2388.

Beresford, H.R. (1978), "Cognitive death: differential problems, Quinlan: Commentary and legal overtones", *Ann. N.Y. Acad. Science*, vol. 315, pp. 339-345.

Brierley, J.B., Adam, J.A.H., Graham, D.I. and Simpson, J.A. (1971), "Neocortical death after cardiac arrest", *Lancet*, vol. ii, pp. 560-565.

Conference of Medical Royal Colleges and their Faculties in the United Kingdom. (1976), "Diagnosis of brain death", *Brit. Med. J.*, vol. 2, pp. 1187-1188.

Conference of Medical Royal Colleges and their Faculties in the United Kingdom. (1979), "Diagnosis of brain death", *Brit. Med. J.*, vol. 1, p. 332.

Cranford, R.E. (1978), "Minnesota Medical Association criteria. Brain death. Concept and criteria", *Minnesota Med.*, vol. 61(9), pp. 561-563. See also: Cranford, R.E. (1978), "Brain death. Concept and criteria", *Minnesota Med.*, vol. 61(10), pp. 600-603.

Cranford, R.E. and Smith, D.R. (1988), "Consciousness: the most critical moral (constitutional) standard for human personhood", *Am. J. Law and Med.*, vol. 13, pp. 233-248.

Evans, M. (1990), "A plea for the heart", *Bioethics*, vol. 4(3), pp. 227-231.

Fackler, J.C. and Rogers, M.C. (1987), "Is brain death really cessation of all intracranial function?", *J. Paediatrics*, vol. 110, pp. 84-86.

Frame, L. (1995), "My little girl dies three times a week", *The Sun*, 8 March, pp. 1-2.

Gervais, K.G. (1986), *Redefining death*. Yale Univ. Press, New Haven, pp. 223-229.

Green, M. and Wickler, D. (1980), "Brain death and personal identity", *Philosophy and Public Affairs*, vol. 9(2), pp. 105-133.

Hall, G.M., Mashiter, K., Lumley, J. and Robson, J.G. (1980), "Hypothalamic pituitary function in the "brain dead" patient", *Lancet* vol. 2, p. 1259.

Hill, D.J. (1987), "Lower oesophageal activity as an indicator of brain death in paralysed and mechanically ventilated patients with head injury", *Brit. Med. J.*, vol. 294, p. 1488.

Jennett, B. and Plum, F. (1972), "Persistent vegetative state after brain damage", *Lancet*, vol. i, p. 734.

Jonas, H. (1974a), "Against the stream: comments on the definition and redefinition of death", in H. Jonas, *Philosophical Essays. From ancient creed to technological man*, Prentice Hall, Englewood Cliffs, pp. 132-140.

Jonas, H. (1974b), "Against the stream: comments on the definition and redefinition of death", in H. Jonas, *Philosophical Essays. From ancient creed to technological man*, Prentice Hall, Englewood Cliffs, p. 130.

Korein, J.L. (1978), "Brain death: terminology, definitions and usage", *Ann.N.Y. Acad. Science*, vol. 315, pp. 6-10.
Lamb, D. (1985), *Death, brain dead and ethics*, Croom Helm, London, p. 139.
Levin, S.D. and Whyte, R.K. (1988), "Brain death sans frontières", *New England J. Med.*, vol. 318, p. 852.
Lynn, J. (1981), "Guidelines for the determination of death. Report of the medical consultants on the diagnosis of death to the President's Commission for the study of ethical problems in medicine and biomedical and behavioural research", *J. American Med. Ass.*, vol. 246, pp. 2184-2186.
McCullagh, P.J. (1993a), *Brain dead, brain absent, brain donors*, John Wiley & Sons Ltd, England, p. 13.
McCullagh, P.J. (1993b), *Brain dead, brain absent, brain donors*, John Wiley & Sons Ltd, England, pp. 14-20.
McCullagh, P.J. (1993c), *Brain dead, brain absent, brain donors*, John Wiley & Sons Ltd, England, p. 14.
McCullagh, P.J. (1993d), *Brain dead, brain absent, brain donors*, John Wiley & Sons Ltd, England, pp. 16-7.
McCullagh, P.J. (1993e), *Brain dead, brain absent, brain donors*, John Wiley & Sons Ltd, England, p. 21.
New York Times. (1976), "Life support ended, a woman dies", *New York Times*, 5 December.
Pallis, C. (1983), *The ABC of brain stem death*, British Medical Assoc., London.
Pallis, C. (1985), "Defining death", *Brit. Med. J.*, vol. 291, pp. 666-667.
Pucetti, R. "Does anyone survive neocortical death?", in R.M. Zaner (ed.), *Beyond whole brain criteria*, Kluwer Academic Publishers, Boston, pp. 75-80.
Robertson, K.M., Hramiak, I.M. and Gelb, A.W. (1989), "Endocrine changes and haemodynamic stability after brain death", *Transplant Proceedings*, vol. 21, pp. 1197-1198.
Schrader, H., Krogness, K., Aakvaag, A., Sortland, O. and Purvis, K. "Changes of pituitary hormones in brain death", *Acta Neurochirurgica*, vol. 52, pp. 239-248.
Sinclair, M.E. (1987), "Lower oesophageal activity as an indicator of brain death in paralysed and mechanically ventilated patients with head injury", *Brit. Med. J.*, vol. 294, p. 1488.
Sweet, W.H. (1978), "Brain death", *New Eng. J. Med.*, vol. 299, pp. 410-412.
Toole, J.F. (1971), "The neurologist and the concept of brain death", *Perspectives in Biology and Medicine*, vol. 14, pp. 599-607.
Veatch, R.M. (1975), "The whole brain oriented concept of death: an outmoded philosophical formulation", *J. Thanatology*, vol. 3, pp. 13-30.
Veatch, R.M. (1989), *Death, dying and the biological revolution*, Yale Univ. Press, New Havèn.
Walton, D.N. (1983), *Ethics of withdrawal of life support systems*, Praeger, New York (reprinted 1987, version referred to), p. 82.
Wetzel, R.C., Setzer, N., Stiff, J.L. and Rogers, M.C. (1985), "Haemodynamic responses in brain dead organ donor patients", *Anaesthesia and Analgesia*, vol. 64, pp. 125-128.
Zaner, R.M. (1988), "Brains and persons: a critique of Veatch's view", in R.M. Zaner (ed.), *Death: beyond whole brain criteria*, Kluwer Academic, Boston, pp. 187-197.

3 Is There a Difference Between Those Declared "Brain Dead" and Those in Persistent Vegetative State or Other Abnormal Brain States?

> *"The dead which are already dead more than the living which are yet alive"*
> Ecclesiastes ch. 4, v. 2

Introduction

It would be useful, if not imperative, to clarify at the beginning exactly what is meant by the various terms in the question and, in addition, to delineate the various other abnormal brain states under consideration. There is an obvious distinction in relation to altered brain states between those altered states containing the term "dead" or "death" and those states that do not contain such a term, *e.g.* persistent vegetative state. This distinction derives from our common, everyday layman's appreciation of the meaning of the term "dead" or "death"; these terms when used by a layman, however, may not always have the same meaning as the same terms used by a member of the medical profession. In addition, arguments have been put forward in the philosophical literature (Gervais, 1976; Veatch, 1989; Beecher, 1968) that some of the states that contain neither of the terms "dead" or "death" should be viewed as being equivalent to those states containing one of these terms. Similarly, an argument has been published taking the stance that the terms "dead" and "death" do not imply permanence of that state (Cole, 1992); this is, obviously, at variance with the common conception of what it means to be dead. With these matters in mind, there seems a strong case for clarification of these various terms and a discussion of what is meant, in physiological terms, by the various altered brain states mentioned earlier.

Abnormal Brain States

There are many altered states of the brain that are considered abnormal, but there is a useful subdivision into those states associated with alteration in consciousness and those in which consciousness is intact (Plum and Posner, 1980). I shall deal firstly with those states associated with an altered level of consciousness.

Delirium

Delirium is a floridly abnormal mental state characterised by disorientation, fear, irritability, misperception of sensory stimuli and, often, visual hallucinations. The behaviour of persons in this state commonly places them completely out of contact with the environment and it is often difficult to determine whether they even retain self-recognition. Lucid periods can alternate with episodes of delirium and during these lucid periods such persons are commonly terrified of their own mental failure. Delirium accompanies diffuse metabolic and multifocal cerebral illnesses and rarely lasts longer than 4-7 days.

Coma

Coma is a state of unrousable unresponsiveness in which the affected person lies with eyes closed. No response to external stimuli or internal need (*e.g.* food) is demonstrated and no sound is uttered.

Vegetative State

Vegetative state is the term proposed by Jennett and Plum (1972) to describe the subacute or chronic condition that sometimes emerges after severe brain injury and comprises a return of wakefulness accompanied by an apparent total lack of cognition. Such patients maintain normal levels of blood pressure and respiratory control. No sounds are uttered although the eyes open in response to verbal stimuli and sleep-wake cycles are established. Persistent or chronic vegetative state refers to this condition in its permanent form (Plum and Posner, 1980) and designates subjects who survive for prolonged periods (sometimes years) without ever recovering any outward manifestations of higher mental function. The term "vegetative state" focuses on the contrast between the severe mental loss and the subject's preserved autonomic or vegetative functions. Several other terms have been invoked to describe the condition of patients in the vegetative state including *coma vigil*, the *apallic syndrome, cerebral death, neocortical death* and *total dementia*. Although these terms may denote minor differences in clinical appearance, all these descriptions apply to a state in which sleeping and waking behaviour have returned to a subject who lacks all evidence of cognition. The neuropathological basis of the persistent vegetative state is well described by Brierley, Adams and Graham (1971). All the brains of the patients studied invariably showed damage to forebrain structures with cortical necrosis sometimes so extensive as to approach total decortication, *i.e.* total loss of the cerebral cortex of the brain. Striking in all the cases was the sparing of brainstem structures. While Korein (1978) has defined cerebral death as "irreversible destruction of both cerebral hemispheres exclusive of the brainstem and cerebellum" and has differentiated it from brain death (see later) the term "cerebral death" is ambiguous because, as Korein himself points out, it has been used by many neurologists as a synonym for brain death, even appearing as such in the literature (Korein, 1978). The term "vegetative state" does not allow for confusion in this respect and will be used in preference to the term "cerebral death". More recently, the term "neocortical death" has been introduced; while it does not have the problem in terms of confusion with brain death, the term "vegetative state" will be preferred, as will be discussed later.

Akinetic Mutism

Akinetic mutism describes a condition of silent alert-appearing immobility associated with sleep-wake cycles. External evidence for mental activity (apart from the appearance of being alert) is absent and spontaneous motor activity is absent. The best clinical and pathological evidence indicates that the classic appearance of akinetic mutism can arise with lesions that interfere with reticular-cortical or limbic-cortical integration but largely spare corticospinal pathways.

Locked-in Syndrome

Locked-in syndrome describes a state in which selective supranuclear motor de-efferentation produces paralysis of all four extremities and the lower cranial nerves without interfering with consciousness. The voluntary motor paralysis prevents the subject from communicating by word or body movement. Usually, but not always, locked-in patients are left with the capacity to use vertical eye movements and blinking to communicate their awareness of internal and external stimuli. Although clinically it somewhat resembles akinetic mutism because of the motor paralysis, and is therefore sometimes confused with it, a "locked-in" patient gives signs of being appropriately aware of himself and the environment, whereas in akinetic mutism little or no awareness appears to exist. Patients chronically in the locked-in state have been taught to signal by Morse code with their eyes and have been able to communicate complex ideas (Feldman, 1971).

Brain Death

Brain death is a state in which all functions of the brain including cortical, subcortical and brainstem functions are permanently lost. Brain death occurs when irreversible brain damage is so extensive that the organ has no potential for recovery and can no longer maintain the body's internal homeostasis, *i.e.* normal respiratory or cardiovascular function, normal temperature control, normal fluid balance control and so on. This state does not require the death of every cell in the brain, but only death of sufficient numbers of cells to abolish function and to render recovery impossible. This apparently simple formulation has been subdivided by the medical profession (and thereafter by philosophers) into cerebral death (or neocortical death or vegetative state) as discussed earlier and brainstem death. This latter is the presently accepted formulation of brain death in the UK, and it is appropriate that it be discussed in some depth.

Brainstem death is a state in which all functions of the brainstem are permanently lost. Total destruction of the brainstem will necessarily entail the permanent cessation of the body's ability to breathe, which in turn deprives the heart and cerebral hemispheres of oxygen thereby causing them to cease functioning. Whilst extensive damage to the cerebral cortex, from trauma or hypoxia, may not cause permanent unconsciousness there is one structure without which consciousness cannot exist. This is the ascending reticular activating system (ARAS) which is situated in the brainstem. Lesions in the brainstem in the areas known as the mesencephalic and pontine tegmentum produce irreversible coma. Hence survival of the brainstem is needed to provide consciousness and breathing. Pallis (1983) has described brainstem death as the "physiological kernel" of brain death. It should be noted that there is nothing intrinsic to the concept of brainstem death that precludes the "higher centres" of the brain from working, since it is implicit in the definition of brainstem death that areas of the brain outwith the brainstem could be normal. Under these circumstances there would not, of course, be any possibility of consciousness but other functions such as temperature control and fluid balance regulation would be intact. (I shall return to a deeper discussion of this topic later in this chapter.)

From the somewhat technical descriptions given above of various altered brain states, it should be obvious that, if a discussion of the ethical and philosophical problems surrounding the concept of brain death is to be undertaken, then the states of coma, persistent vegetative state, akinetic mutism, locked-in syndrome in addition to brain death (and its subdivisions) are the states that are of interest. It would be worthwhile to reiterate what has been said in plain, layman's terms because it is my opinion that much of the confusion (and, consequently, the arguments) about brain death and other associated states is a result of incomplete understanding of the meaning of the terms used to describe the various states. Coma is a state of unconsciousness in which there is no apparent response to stimuli of any description; the term has been used to describe the state existing in the persistent vegetative state but this is not accurate in that a person in coma does not develop "sleep-wake cycles". That is, a patient in coma does not exhibit periods of time when the eyes are closed alternating with periods of time when the eyes are open and, perhaps, roving around although not fixing on any one object and not showing any evidence of cognition; there is no evidence of consciousness. The appearance of the "sleep-wake cycle", is found in the persistent vegetative state, but again there is no evidence of cognition. Also found in the persistent vegetative state but not necessarily in coma is the ability to maintain homeostasis, *i.e.* the ability to maintain the integrity of the body as a whole; some patients in coma may demonstrate this ability but this I feel illustrates the rather vague definition of the term "coma" and the consequent confusion that arises from such vagueness of definition. I feel that the term "coma" is best avoided for this reason.

Other terms have become synonymous with the persistent vegetative state, *viz.* cerebral death and neocortical death. Both of these former terms contain precise anatomical terms and it should be made clear what they mean and, more, importantly, how they differ. The term "cerebral death" implies the death of the cerebrum (or cerebral hemisphere). The cerebral hemispheres form the largest part of the brain and the term includes all structures from the surface of that part of the brain to deep, midline structures such as the wall of the third ventricle and all intermediately placed structures such as the basal nuclei (Warwick and Williams, 1973). I have already alluded to the confusion that has arisen in the literature between the terms "cerebral death" and "brain death"; this is sufficient reason for not using the former term. However, the use of the term "cerebral death" synonymously with the terms "neocortical death" and "persistent vegetative state" is another matter and merits some discussion. Having discussed the anatomical meaning of the term "cerebrum" it is relevant to contrast that with the anatomical structures included in the term "neocortical". This latter term refers to the cerebral cortex, a structure that is a mantle covering the cerebral hemisphere and variable in thickness (1.5 to 4.5 mm (Warwick and Williams, 1973)). It should now be obvious that the cerebral cortex or neocortex is only a part (a small part) of the whole cerebral hemisphere; it follows that the terms "cerebral death" and "neocortical death" are not synonymous since the former term implies death of much more brain tissue than does the latter. It may be argued that these anatomical differences are not entirely relevant since the clinical picture produced by both conditions, *i.e.* cerebral death and neocortical death, are identical. However, careful examination of the differences in anatomical tissue affected reveals that this is not the case. In cerebral death, all the deep structures of the cerebral hemisphere would be functionally lost, whereas in the state of neocortical death these deep structures would be left functionally intact. One example to demonstrate this difference would be that in cerebral death the nuclei with connections to the pituitary gland would cease to function with consequent loss of pituitary function; in neocortical death these nuclei would remain functioning and the pituitary gland would continue to function normally. The clinical result of this would be that in cerebral death there would be loss of the ability to control fluid and electrolyte balance, whereas this same function would be intact in the state of neocortical death. Hence the two terms "cerebral death" and "neocortical death" are not synonymous. It also follows from my immediately preceding comments that the terms "cerebral death" and "persistent vegetative state" are not synonymous since in the persistent vegetative state normal pituitary function is retained and there is no loss of fluid balance control. Hence the term "cerebral death", is not synonymous with either the term "neocortical death" or the term "persistent vegetative state". Finally, the relationship between the terms "neocortical death" and "persistent vegetative state" has to be examined. As I discussed earlier, the term "neocortical death" implies the death of the cortex of the cerebral hemispheres and this corresponds very closely to the pathological findings described by Brierley *et al* (1971) in their cases of established persistent vegetative state. The term also implies that other areas in the brain are intact and this feature is, again, an invariable finding reported by these authors. This empirical evidence supports the view that the neuropathological term "neocortical death" is certainly consistent with the clinical condition of persistent vegetative state, and supports the argument that the two terms are equivalent. It should be remembered, however, that "neocortical death" is a neuropathological term, whereas "persistent vegetative state" is a descriptive term applied to a clinical condition; it may be possible that the clinical condition can be produced as a result of pathological processes other than neocortical death. Hence, while the term "neocortical death" can be considered equivalent to "persistent vegetative state", it does not necessarily follow that the reverse is true or that "persistent vegetative state" is always equivalent to "neocortical death". For this reason, I prefer to use the term "persistent vegetative state" (PVS), since I am primarily concerned with the clinical condition and not necessarily with the underlying neuropathological process.

The discussion now turns to the condition of the locked-in syndrome (LIS). This condition is classically caused by vascular insults to the brainstem or by infection; in the latter case, the LIS is generally temporary. The unfortunate person in this condition is totally unable to move any limb and requires artificial ventilation; the only movement possible is that of blinking the eyes. It has been well described by survivors of the temporary form produced by extremely severe forms of the Guillain-Barré syndrome as having a brain and a mind completely unattached to any physical body, since no movement is possible, but, at the same time, being totally dependent on the physical body and the care given to that body by attendants. Such patients are always conscious and aware of the environment (assuming that there is no other pathological process producing impediment to this awareness). In addition, if good communication can be established, it becomes obvious that there is no intellectual impairment and that the "higher" functions of the brain are intact. The condition of the locked-in syndrome can be confused with the much rarer condition of akinetic mutism. In this latter state, there is no apparent evidence to indicate that there is any mental activity unlike the locked-in syndrome in which evidence for such activity is only too apparent once communication has been established. In other respects, the two conditions produce similar clinical appearances. Perhaps as a result of the rarity of the locked-in syndrome it has been overlooked in the literature on brain death and the two quite separate conditions have, on occasion, been confused and conflated. This is understandable in the lay press, but in academic discussion about brain death and allied disordered brain states, it is imperative that any such confusion be avoided. A comparison between PVS and LIS at this stage would be instructive, and a comparison between those two conditions and brain death will be discussed later after discussion of the latter condition has been completed. The problem with PVS and LIS is that both conditions appear to present with an unconscious person and it is this superficial similarity that, in my opinion, has led to confusion; a person in PVS is unconscious but a person in LIS is most definitely not unconscious and, indeed, such a person (in LIS) is fully conscious and able to communicate albeit in a limited fashion. Secondly, all patients in LIS require artificial ventilation, whereas patients in PVS do not require such intervention and, indeed, are able to maintain not only their own breathing but also all the regulatory mechanisms associated with spontaneous breathing. It should be obvious that the two conditions of PVS and LIS are not the same.

The term "brain death" describes a state in which there has been permanent loss of all brain function including cortical, subcortical and brainstem function. The result of this is irreversible unconsciousness and permanent loss of the ability to maintain the body's normal homeostasis; such a patient is unable to breathe and requires artificial ventilation. In addition, there would be, in such a patient, hypothermia and profound fluid and electrolyte loss as a result of the loss of function of the hypothalamus and pituitary gland; the combination of these two deficits, if not treated, usually results in cardiac instability and asystole in a matter of hours. It can be seen, therefore, that the condition of brain death is an accurate predictor of the appearance of the two classical findings of death, *viz.* lack of breathing and lack of heartbeat. If these systemic disturbances can be corrected and maintained, normal cardiac function can be maintained for some time although, ultimately, asystole supervenes (Pallis, 1983). This should be contrasted with PVS in which cardiac function and breathing are normal and remain under the control of the patient (although there is no voluntary control of these functions); permanent unconsciousness is the one feature common to brain death and PVS.

Earlier in this chapter, I indicated that whilst brainstem death produced permanent unconsciousness and inability to breathe, other functions of the brain would be intact since there was nothing in the term "brainstem death" to imply any dysfunction of other areas of the brain. The problem that my description of brainstem death differs markedly from what is met with in clinical practice is one that I should address. I have suggested that the term "brainstem death" does not indicate anything about the functional status of the remainder of the brain, and I would hold the view that my description of brainstem death as detailed above is a valid one. The clinical picture of brainstem death commonly met with is not merely a picture of brainstem death but also includes features that indicate that other areas of the brain are not working, *e.g.* it is often found that a massive diuresis occurs in brainstem death. This certainly happens but it is not as a result of brainstem death but as a result of dysfunction and perhaps death of the hypothalamus. Thus the diuresis may be temporally related to brainstem death but not causally related to it. It is for this reason that the clinical picture of brainstem death does not match the description that I have given earlier. It is possible that the appearances of brainstem death are mimicked by other conditions that do not affect consciousness, and that, simultaneously, the patient suffers from a second, reversible, condition that adversely affects consciousness; such a coincidence is not as unlikely as first appears if one considers that the majority of patients with brain death or brainstem death have suffered cranial trauma and may be unconscious for a variety of reasons not immediately connected with the cranial trauma, *e.g.* drugs or alcohol. One scenario that raises the possibility of misdiagnosis of brainstem death is a patient with severe Guillain-Barré disease. This condition, which is usually temporary but which can be permanent, produces a transverse myelitis of the spinal cord, abolishing all function below that point; occasionally, this process ascends up the cord to the brainstem resulting in total loss of brainstem function. This state, *per se*, would not be mistaken for brainstem death by any competent clinician because such a patient would be expected to be conscious as opposed to the brainstem dead patient who would be unconscious. However, let us consider a case of unusually severe Guillain-Barré disease in which loss of function of the facial and eye muscles occurred and this loss appeared to be permanent (there is no pathophysiological reason why this particular clinical condition should not occur). Consider this scenario carefully; this patient would be conscious but unable to move limbs, face or eyes, would require artificial ventilation and would have been in this condition for some considerable time (in order to allow the term "permanent" reasonably to be used in light of the known natural history of Guillain-Barré disease). In such a case, misinterpretation of the clinical signs could lead to the misdiagnosis of brainstem death and potentially inappropriate treatment. However, these are rare conditions and it could be argued that such errors would be extremely rare in clinical practice. However, errors in classification occur outwith medical practice and such mistakes may lead to errors in argument when they occur in the philosophical literature (Jonas, 1974; Evans, 1990) or to potential mistakes in judgement when they occur in the legal profession (Lord Edmund-Davies, 1977; Williams, 1973; Skegg, 1974). It is important, therefore, to appreciate the distinct conditions and the different clinical states associated with each.

It is appropriate at this point to address the question of the differences between the state referred to as "brain death" and the other altered brain states. One immediate and obvious difference is the use of the term "death" in the nomenclature of certain states, *viz.* brain death, brainstem death, neocortical death and cerebral death. (I am aware that I have already stated that I do not like this latter term, but I have included it here partly for completeness and partly because it helps to demonstrate my point.) The one feature common to all the states in which the term "death" appears is that of unconsciousness, *i.e.* all the altered brain states that are commonly referred to in terms containing the term "death" have unconsciousness as one of their features. However, the use of the term "death" in these circumstances is as a pathological descriptor linked to an anatomical term, *e.g.* brain death or neocortical death. There is nothing implicit in the use of the term, *i.e.* death, under these circumstances that would indicate that the organism as a whole should have the same term applied to it. The term in these cases is being used as an indicator that an anatomical structure is permanently non-functional. However, I think that it is significant that the only states that are so described are those that are associated with unconsciousness and that we do not describe the locked-in syndrome in its permanent form (which can be produced as a result of non-recovery from severe Guillain-Barré disease or from an unusual form of "stroke") as "partial brainstem death" although that would be a neuropathologically correct descriptive term. It would seem that we reserve the use of the term "death" in relation to the description of altered brain states exclusively for those states that are associated with permanent unconsciousness. This, I would suggest, is a reflection of the importance that is placed upon consciousness by the majority of observers. This importance is best illustrated by the arguments put forward by Gervais (1976), Beecher (1968), Veatch (1989) and Pucetti (1988) that those in whom consciousness has been permanently lost should be viewed as dead. It is, probably, no accident that there is this close association between unconsciousness and the use of the term "death" in the description of some altered brain states. This association does not help with the question of the differences between brain death and the other altered brain states, since it does not adequately separate brain death from *all* the other states, although it does separate brain death from *some* of the other states, *e.g.* locked-in syndrome and akinetic mutism.

Another feature of brain death in addition to unconsciousness that is common to some of the other altered brain states is the loss of the ability to maintain breathing. It is pertinent, at this point, to clarify some terms that are in common use in the literature on brain death and allied topics. The terms breathing and ventilation are not interchangeable; breathing is a spontaneous event initiated by the person himself and cannot be performed for him by another person (mouth-to-mouth resuscitation) or by mechanical means (artificial ventilators). Ventilation is the term applied to what is done by others or by mechanical means to those who are unable to breathe. What is lost in brain death and some of the other altered brain states is the ability to breathe because the central mechanism required to drive the peripheral apparatus of breathing is no longer functioning. The conditions that have this as a feature are the locked-in syndrome, brain death and brainstem death, all other altered states leaving the victim with the ability to breathe. However, severe Guillain-Barré syndrome may also result in the loss of the ability to breathe by one of two possible mechanisms. If the disease affects only the cervical spinal cord, the cord in this area will not conduct the signals arising in the brainstem and the victim will not breathe; the second mechanism comes into play when the disease affects the brainstem itself, resulting in the loss of the ability to generate the signals required to initiate breathing. This latter mechanism is similar to the loss of signal generation in brain death and brainstem death and may be similarly permanent. Two conditions not previously discussed that are similar to the first mechanism (in relation to Guillain-Barré syndrome) are polio and cervical cord injury. In both of these conditions, the cervical cord cannot transmit the signals it receives from the intact brainstem and the end result is the inability to breathe. It seems to me that the exact mechanism whereby the ability to breathe is lost is relatively unimportant. Whether or not a person has permanently lost the ability to breathe because of brainstem death, locked-in syndrome or one of the other conditions discussed above, *i.e.* severe Guillain-Barré disease, polio and cervical spinal cord injury, is not relevant to the more important question of the moral status of that person. That is, the question of whether or not a person is dead cannot rest solely on that person's ability to breathe. (Pallis argues that the question of whether or not a person is dead could, however, rest on this loss of the ability to breathe *plus* some specific cause for the loss of this ability (Pallis, 1983).)

If we examine what I have explored so far, it is obvious that I have failed to demonstrate that there is a single property or collection of properties that pertain only to the state of brain death. Examining the previous paragraphs, it is obvious that I have not isolated a feature that *per se* distinguishes brain death from the other abnormal brain states under discussion. Even if we amalgamate the features we have discussed, *viz.* apnoea and unconsciousness, we find that while these conditions certainly exist in the state of brain death, it is possible that they could also exist in any of the other altered brain states if there were also concomitant cervical spinal cord injury—a set of circumstances that is by no means unlikely. It is possible, therefore, that some of the other altered brain states, if co-existing with, for example cervical spinal cord injury, could mimic brain death. It is, therefore, unlikely that a collection of features which include one or more features that can be produced other than by brain dysfunction will determine (or be used to determine) the difference between brain death and the other altered brain states. An objection could be raised here that the difficulties that I cite are practical rather than conceptual difficulties. My reply would be to argue that in order that the criteria and tests for death cannot be mistaken for signs of other, non-fatal, disorders, the concept of death must be such that the criteria derived from it and the tests for death derived in turn from the criteria, cannot be duplicated or mimicked by other non-fatal disease. The feature or features that could be used as such a determinant should reside in or depend upon an intact brain and not the peripheral nervous system or any other physiological system. Perhaps the clue to a potential feature is in the term itself. The term "brain death" implies the death of the brain as a whole and this is quite different from all the other states under discussion that include the term "death"; these latter states have permanent non-function of only part of the brain. It is possible, therefore, to approach the question of the possible difference between brain death and the other altered brain states from another route.

Let us examine the possibility that there is another feature, not yet discussed, that may distinguish brain death from all the other abnormal brain states and that belongs to brain death as a direct result of the fact that the whole brain, as an organ, has died. To help in this approach, it would be useful to examine the anatomical structures that are rendered permanently inoperative in brain death but which remain functional in the other states.

The major anatomical difference between brain death and the other states is the involvement, in brain death only, of the midline structures, *viz.* the thalamus and hypothalamus; these are not affected in the other states and function normally. The normal function of the hypothalamus is to regulate temperature, fluid balance, acid-base balance and blood pressure; in addition there is also control of heart rate and initiation and control of breathing. These functions are collectively referred to as homeostasis, *i.e.* maintenance of the internal environment of the body. These functions are intact in all the other altered brain states but are permanently lost in brain death, because the necessary anatomical structures are unaffected in the other brain states but permanently non-functioning in brain death. This, then, is the property that is uniquely lost in brain death; only in the state of brain death is the control of homeostasis lost. The next question is, of course, whether or not this property of control of homeostasis is important. This question can be answered on two levels, the physiological and the philosophical. At present, I will answer it briefly at the physiological level; the question is raised again and discussed in greater depth in chapters 6 and 7. What we are really asking here is whether or not homeostasis is physiologically important to an organism. If we accept that homeostasis is the maintenance of the internal environment in terms of temperature, fluid composition and pH then there can be no doubt that homeostasis is vitally important for the continued existence of the organism. Empirical observation shows that organisms (including humans) stressed beyond the limits of the control of homeostasis or whose normal homeostatic controls have been abolished, do not survive. There can be no doubt that in terms of physiology the ability to control homeostasis is of paramount importance. Once the control of homeostasis has been lost, the cells of the organism are merely "running down" in terms of the energy normally contained in them and needed for essential processes such as maintenance of the cell membrane, *i.e.* the maintenance of their physical integrity. This physiological question and answer are, of course, different from any philosophical question about the rôle of the control of homeostasis. What is important from the philosophical point of view is the answer to the question "When is the organism dead?" This latter point, I would contend, is the point at which control of homeostasis is lost and this topic is explored in depth in chapter 10.

Earlier, I discussed the importance of breathing in relation to brain death, persistent vegetative state and the locked-in syndrome and I would like, at this point, to turn to the question of the rôle of the beating heart in brain death and the altered brain states and contrast it with the rôle of breathing. In all the conditions discussed, the heart beats spontaneously unlike breathing which is lost in several states, *e.g.* brain death, brain stem death and the locked-in syndrome. It would seem from this that the presence of a spontaneously beating heart cannot be a determinant in the classification and separation of these states. However, it would seem that the presence of a spontaneously beating heart is a barrier to some (Jonas, 1974; Evans, 1990) who would maintain that death cannot be viewed as having occurred until the heart stops beating. Certainly the traditional criteria for death have been (and still are) the cessation of breathing and the cessation of the heartbeat, but it is essential to contrast these two physiological phenomena because although they are frequently paired together, they are significantly different in their relationship with the central nervous system. Breathing, as I have indicated earlier in this paper, is a spontaneous activity but relies for this spontaneity on connections to the brain; if these connections are rendered inoperative either by disruption of the peripheral nerves (phrenic nerve and the intercostal nerves), malfunction of the cervical spinal cord or the brainstem, then breathing ceases. Not only is breathing controlled in its depth and rate by the brainstem, but the very act of breathing is initiated by the brainstem; in other words, disconnection from the brainstem for whatever reason results not merely in a reduction in the rate or depth of breathing but in the total cessation of breathing. Consider now the rôle of the central nervous system with respect to the beating heart. In the intact organism, the spontaneous heartbeat is actually the result of a complex interplay between the heart muscle and the connections to the central nervous system and differs significantly from breathing. Several physiological facts should be borne in mind with respect to cardiac muscle and the connections to the central nervous system. Cardiac muscle contracts ("beats") spontaneously or intrinsically without any connection to the central nervous system. The evidence for this is twofold. Firstly there are the empirical observations in embryology that indicate that the foetal heart in the human begins to beat at approximately 4 weeks of gestation before any neural connections have reached it (and, incidentally, prior to the formation of the vascular system) (Warwick and Williams, 1973). The second empirical observation is from routine physiological experiments in which a heart can be removed from an organism and placed in a container with saline and some nutrients; such a totally enervated heart will continue to beat for some hours or even days if close control is exerted over the supply of nutrients. That the heart can beat spontaneously without any central neural connections is beyond doubt. So what, then, is the rôle of the well-documented central neural connections?

The function of these is to control heart function and "fine-tune" it to the requirements of the organism; in other words, the central neural connections are responsible for controlling the rate of the heartbeat and the stroke volume of each beat (*i.e.* the volume pumped out with each beat). Without functioning central neural connections, the heart returns to its intrinsic rate of beating of approximately 30-35 beats per minute and to a much reduced stroke volume; this state is barely compatible with consciousness and most patients precipitated into this state by acute heart disease become unconscious. It is for this reason that in cardiac transplantation the all-important sino-atrial node of the recipient's heart is retained; without this node that is essentially the point of connection of the nerves from the central nervous system with the heart, the donor heart when transplanted would remain at its intrinsic rhythm and be of very little, if any, use to the recipient. Therefore, a spontaneously beating heart in the absence of central neural connections (and thereby outwith the control of the brain) is merely a demonstration of the physiological properties of cardiac muscle and is of no use to the intact organism.

Let us consider an analogy between the body and a central heating system, and use this to illustrate the rôle of the heart and also perhaps to clarify the differences between brain death and the other altered brain states. The components of the central heating system (with suggested organic equivalents in brackets) are:

- boiler (lungs);
- pump (heart);
- radiator (cells of body);
- controller ("vegetative" part of brain/brainstem and hypothalamus);
- temperature sensor ("vegetative" part of brain/brainstem and hypothalamus);
- rooms of house in which central heating is situated ("higher" functions of brain); while this is not, in strict terms, part of a central heating system, it has been included here because it sheds some light on the later explanations.

There is one difference from a normal central heating system that I must impose upon the analogy and that is that the pump runs continually and that the controller only alters its rate but cannot shut it down; this is to allow the pump to more closely resemble its organic counterpart the heart which, as I have explained earlier in this chapter, beats spontaneously but whose rate and stroke volume are controlled by the brainstem. Let us also assume that the controller is normally timed, *i.e.* it will start and stop the system at pre-determined times, but that this can be over-ridden by the sensor (a normal arrangement in central heating systems).

Under normal circumstances, all the components of the central heating system are working, the controller switching the system on and off and intermittently being over-ridden by the external sensor; the boiler is used as needed to maintain the temperature and the pump works continuously, but when needed the pump rate can be increased by the controller to deal with sudden fluctuations in temperature detected by the external sensor. In the organic model under normal circumstances, the brainstem and the hypothalamus run the body and allow sleep-wake cycles, the lungs and the heart run continuously with the rate of each being varied by the controller as the demand for alteration is assessed by the sensor. Let us examine at this analogy under different circumstances.

In the state of *brain death*, in which we would lose the controller, sensor and boiler we would be left with a system in which the pump would continue to work at its intrinsic rate but would be pumping cold water since the boiler would not function. In addition, the rooms have become uninhabitable as a result of the lack of heat. If the boiler were supported externally then the water moved by the pump would be warm (as the blood is oxygenated when artificial ventilation is performed to support breathing that has failed), but this would not alter the fact that all internal control of the system had been permanently lost. An important difference between biological and non-biological systems needs to be stressed here. In non-biological systems, a system breakdown can be analysed and repaired at will. This is not the case in biological systems in which a breakdown in the system will result not only in the system not working but also, and importantly, in the system beginning to be "taken apart" as the energy required for maintenance of the components of the biological system falls below a critical level. The result of this difference is that there is a crucial time after which a biological system cannot be restarted as the components of the system are no longer physically intact.

In the *locked-in syndrome*, the rooms of the house would be intact (higher brain functions intact) but the controller and sensor would be partially lost with resultant loss of control of the boiler (lungs) and pump (heart). Hence, in this state, higher mental functions such as abstract thoughts could continue but only if the rest of the system could be supported by external means. It is true that the sensor would have no control over this external support system, but that may be a reflection of our technological ability to combine biological and non-biological systems into a complete coherent whole. If this latter step could be achieved, then a person in the locked-in syndrome would be capable of independent existence that would, at the same time, be under his or her control. This state would not be too different from the "normal" state enjoyed by the same person prior to the event that deprived him/her of the ability to control his/her own system. In view of my previous comments earlier in this chapter about brainstem death, *viz.* that there is nothing implicit in the term "brainstem death" that implies non-functioning of other areas of the brain, it should be obvious that the sequence of events discussed here in relation to persistent vegetative state could also be applied to brainstem death, namely that external support for the functions lost could be given and a human being who is technically "brainstem dead" could be awake and alert. This state of affairs, of course, could occur only if the external support for the functions lost could be put in place prior to the actual loss of the functions; as I have already indicated, brain death follows brainstem death in a very short space of time and this external support that is theoretically possible is not possible in practice.

In the case of the *persistent vegetative state*, the elements lost would be the rooms of the house (higher mental functions) and nothing else. In other words, the system could continue to function as a system, but without any apparent purpose, that is a central heating system with nothing to heat. It may be asked, in the light of my remarks in the preceding paragraph, whether or not the functions of the rooms could be replaced. Certainly in the central heating system such a procedure would raise no great problems (the rooms could be redesigned or even new rooms built), but this would not be the case in the biological system. If the rooms (that is, the higher mental functions) could be replaced (and it should be borne in mind that this question remains in the realms of philosophical enquiry and science fiction, since there is no prospect of such a procedure being feasible in the foreseeable future) then one is forced to ask questions about the nature of this new system. For example, "Is this system the same as the previous one?" or "Is this new system different from the previous system?" Questions such as these are pertinent when it is remembered that what is being lost when the rooms are lost in PVS is the capacity for higher mental functions. If the replacement "rooms" have different mental functions, then we are entitled to ask if the resultant system is identical to the system it replaces. Replacement of the rooms remains, therefore, in the realm of philosophical speculation and raises serious philosophical questions about the new system. This is not germane to the main thrust of my argument and will not be pursued further.

In the state of *brainstem death*, the rooms for a very short time would be intact (see my earlier discussion of brainstem death in this chapter), but would be permanently lost thereafter, but there would be loss of the controller and thereby loss of control of the boiler and pump; the pump would continue to run but at a low, basal rate without the control from the controller. This state, that is the state of brainstem death when the rooms have been permanently lost differs significantly from the state of the locked-in syndrome and does not differ significantly from the clinical condition of brain death. The essential physiological difference between the locked-in syndrome (LIS) and brainstem death as I have described the latter state is that in the LIS the connections between the brainstem and the cortex remain functioning whereas these connections are lost in brainstem death. In terms of the analogy, LIS has rooms that are normal and a controller that works imperfectly in some of its functions allowing the rooms to function; in brainstem death, the rooms may be working (for a short time) but we cannot detect this because the connections from the controller to the rooms have been lost. This is the subtle, but real, difference between LIS and brainstem death.

Summary

What I have argued so far is that there are differences between the state of brain death, persistent vegetative state and other altered brain states in strict physiological terms. I have suggested that an important physiological function is the ability to control homeostasis and I have argued from empirical data that this ability is lost only in the state of brain death. I will proceed, in later chapters, to argue that the ability to control homeostasis is fundamental to all life and, therefore could be considered as the criterion on which decisions regarding the ontological status of a human being (or other animal) in terms of life could be based.

References

Beecher, H.K. (1968), "A definition of irreversible coma. Report of the *ad hoc* committee of the Harvard Medical School to examine the definition of brain death", *J. American Med. Ass.*, vol. 205, pp. 337-340 (see also Beecher, H.K. (1969), "After the 'definition of irreversible coma'", *New Eng. J. Med*, vol. 281, pp. 1070-1071.)

Brierley, J.B., Adams, J.H., Graham, D.I. and Simpson, J.A. (1971), "Neocortical death after cardiac arrest", *Lancet*, vol. ii, pp. 560-565.

Cole, D.J. (1992), "The reversibility of death", *J. Med. Ethics*, vol. 18, pp. 26-30.

Edmund-Davies, Lord. (1977), "On dying and dying well", *Proc. Roy. Soc. Med*, vol. 70, p. 73.
Evans, M. (1990), "A plea for the heart", *Bioethics*, vol. 4(3), pp. 227-231.
Feldman, M.H. (1971), "Physiological observations in a chronic case of locked-in syndrome", *Neurology*, vol. 21, pp. 459-478.
Gervais, K.G. (1986), *Redefining death*, Yale Univ. Press, New Haven.
Jennett, W.B. and Plum, F. (1972), "Persistent vegetative state after brain damage: a syndrome looking for a name", *Lancet*, vol. i, pp. 734-737.
Jonas, H. (1974), "Against the stream: comments on the definition and redefinition of death", in H. Jonas, *Philosophical essays: from ancient creed to technological man*. Univ. Of Chicago Press, Chicago, (reprinted 1980).
Korein, J. (1978), "Brain death: interrelated medical and social issues", *Ann. N.Y. Acad. Science*, vol. 315, pp. 1-454 (see also Korein, J. (1978), "Brain death: terminology, definitions and usage", *Ann. N.Y. Acad. Science*, vol. 315, pp. 6-10).
Pallis, C. (1983), *The ABC of brainstem death*, British Medical Assoc., London.
Plum, F. and Posner, J.B. (1980), *The diagnosis of stupor and coma*, 3rd ed., F.A. Davis Co., Philadelphia.
Puccetti, R. (1988), "Does anyone survive neocortical death?", in R.M. Zaner (ed.), *Death: beyond whole brain criteria*, Kluwer Academic, Boston, pp. 75-90.
Skegg, P.D. (1974), "Irreversibly comatosed individuals: alive or dead?", *Cambridge Law J*, vol. 33, p. 130.
Veatch, R.M. (1989), *Death, dying and the biological revolution*, Yale Univ. Press, New Haven (see also, Veatch, R.M. (1975), "The whole brain oriented concept of death: an outmoded philosophical formulation", *J. Thanatology*, vol. 3, pp. 13-30).
Warwick, R. and Williams, P.L. (1973), *Gray's Anatomy*, 35th ed., Longman, Edinburgh.
Williams, G. (1973), "Euthanasia", *Med.-Legal J.*, vol. 41, p. 14.

4 Reasons for Rejection of the Present Concepts of Death

"As soon as an idea is accepted it is time to reject it"
Holbrook Jackson *Platitudes in the making* p. 13

Introduction

Again, I would like to return to the quote by Dennett at the beginning of this monograph. It is worth re-iterating that all the concepts of death discussed in this monograph have been chosen and not discovered; arguments have been put forward for all of the concepts to be discussed. However, many of these arguments have developed into dogma and, as a result, the arguments are not critically examined. I agree with Dennett that the dogma surrounding these fundamentally arbitrary attempts is in never-ending need of examination.

General

The general idea of death as commonly understood appears to involve the notion of the loss of something vital. A philosophical understanding of death would bracket this general idea together with a resultant change in ontological status (from "alive" to "dead"). Apart from religious views of death and the afterlife, which would tend to deny the ordinary conception of death or to relocate the importance of death away from bodily destruction, most concepts of death would be negative ones in terms of loss. With regard to the idea that there are necessary conditions of life that are lost in death, it is essential that the condition or conditions of life that are lost be *necessary* conditions and not merely contingent features of life. This requirement that the conditions of life to be lost in the change in ontological status from "alive" to "dead" be necessary ones is essential in order to be able to make a completely exclusive distinction between life and death, that is where death applies, life must be completely excluded; this is guaranteed by the non-meeting of some necessary condition or conditions. From this I wish to defend the proposition that the concept of death concerns a state which stands in absolute contrast with life, in which one or more conditions for life are categorically unmet, and to which one moves by first being alive and then losing life through categorically losing the capacity to meet one or more of those necessary conditions.

Concepts of Death

Many concepts of death have been put forward and some have been in use for many generations as I have outlined in the introduction. Related to these concepts are appropriate criteria and tests to ascertain that the criteria have been met. It follows that any change in the concept of death will necessitate corresponding changes in the criteria and tests for death. It does not follow that any changes in the criteria and tests imply that a change of concept has occurred. Such changes in criteria and tests may indicate only that refinements of previous criteria and tests have been adopted. A commonly quoted example of such a refinement in tests is the introduction of the use of stethoscopes and the electrocardiogram (ECG) in the determination of death; this did not entail any change in the traditional heart-lung based concept of death.

Criteria for death can have meaning only if they can be shown to be logically derived from the appropriate concept of death (Lamb, 1985a). It is meaningless to use "free-floating" criteria that are not logically derived from a clearly determined concept of death (Browne, 1983; Pallis, 1983a). It should also be borne in mind that adequately derived criteria and tests do not necessarily imply that the concept of death, from whence they were derived, is philosophically adequate. An excellent example of this is given by Pallis (1983b):

> " In the Middle Ages, if one entered certain monasteries one ceased to enjoy the limited rights and heavy duties of the outside world. One would be considered "dead" by civil society. The appropriate criteria for such a concept would presumably be a certificate from the Father Superior of the monastery confirming that one had entered it. Esoteric concepts may be met by esoteric criteria."

If we are to accept that we are looking for a concept of death that will be relevant to the "organism as a whole" then we must avoid any vaguely formulated or indeterminate concepts. Thus, a concept of death as "the loss of that which is essentially significant to the nature of man" is unsatisfactory, since we could say that an individual has lost what is essentially significant but is still alive, because concepts like "essentially significant" and "the nature of man" are undetermined. In addition, it is possible to define the term "essentially significant" in more than one way and it would follow that an individual could then be dead by one concept and alive by another; this would be a very unsatisfactory state of affairs. These anomalies arise largely because of the indeterminancy of the terms "essentially significant" and "the nature of man" but also because the features (of the entity) chosen as important for the ontological change from "alive" to "dead" may not be necessary features of life, that is they are not essential for life, but are contingent upon it in some entities. An example of these indeterminate terms is Veatch's (1989a) "capacity for social interaction". The loss of this feature of human life would be unfortunate and unquestionably crippling for the individual concerned, but it would plainly not be fatal. In order to avoid these anomalies, only a concept of death that specifies the irreversible loss of a necessary feature of life should be considered as a concept of death.

One might have various reasons for adopting any given concept of death, but such reasons must include or involve the following:

- The concept explains known events, that is the concept can adequately encompass the death of all humans. The capacity to explain the death of all humans I would view as a minimum essential property of any concept of death. Others may reject the concept because it cannot offer an adequate explanation of the death of animals but that is not my primary concern.
- The arguments for the concept must be convincing.
- The concept should allow formulation of definitions and hence of tests for death since death, while an abstract entity in philosophical discussion, is also a commanding practical problem.

In addition, it would be desirable that the concept be consistent, that is explain events in as many situations as possible: a concept of A that explains A in only a very limited number of circumstances would not be a good or useful concept. In relation to any concept of death, it should be remembered that death is universal to all living entities, including human beings, and it would be desirable that any concept of death should be able to include the deaths of these entities and not be restricted to any one section or group of entities. If one had a concept of death that encompassed only a subgroup of all living entities, then at least one other concept of death would be required for the remaining group or groups not encompassed by the original concept. This would mean that there would be more than one concept of death, that is an event that is universal to all living entities would have more that one concept; not a desirable state of affairs at all. It is desirable that a universal event should have a universal concept.

With these general comments in mind, I will address the problem of the present concepts of death. The current concepts of death have been well discussed by Veatch (1989a) and I will follow his outline.

Irreversible Loss of the Soul from the Body

This is the traditional religious and, until recently, philosophical view in western culture. Essentially, it held that a person died at the time when the soul left the body. This may seem, as it has seemed in the past, to be a reasonable concept of death, but it does not satisfy all of the criteria mentioned above.

Firstly, Christianity takes the view that the soul is an essential element in the living human being, but importantly it also adopted the Aristotelian view that human beings differ from other living creatures in possessing a rational soul in addition to vegetative and animal souls. While this latter concept of the elements of a living human being was later modified, it remains that a living human being has a soul that other animals do not possess. (The position of plants in relation to the possession of souls is not clear.) What is clear, however, is that the concept of death containing the term "soul" will probably not encompass plants or animals other than human beings.

Secondly, the requirement within the concept that the soul leaves the body is a requirement that has proven difficult to verify experimentally and scientifically. No one has directly or indirectly ascertained the moment of the soul leaving the body. Accordingly, criteria cannot be formulated as a logical process from such a concept and, as a result of the lack of criteria, no test (or tests) of death can be derived. Pope Pius, while holding to the traditional view stated above, indicated that the determination of death is best left to the medical profession but did not indicate how this determination of death is, or should be related to the concept of death that he promulgated (Pope Pius, 1957). This lack of criteria and tests severely limit the usefulness of this concept and I would suggest that it is probably best left to the religious traditions.

Another objection to the use of this concept of death, apart from the practical difficulties outlined earlier, is that society is becoming increasingly secular and belief in the existence of the soul is not as widespread as it once was. It would seem unreasonable, under these circumstances, to attempt to conceive of death in terms in which few people believed or to impose that concept of death upon them.

Irreversible Loss of the Flow of Vital Fluids

Religious believers might see the departure of the soul from the body as occurring at about the time that the vital fluids stop flowing, but it would be a mistake to equate these two concepts of death. In the "loss of flow" concept, the fluid stops from natural causes (even if unexplained) and death is nothing more than that cessation of flow, whereas in the "loss of soul" concept the fluids cease to flow at the time the soul departs and it stops because the soul departs. In this latter case, the essential thing is the loss of the soul and not the cessation of the fluid flow.

The "vital fluids" referred to here are commonly understood to be the breath and the blood and this simple and straightforward definition is adequate for my purposes. This movement of liquids and gases at the organismic and cellular levels is a distinguishing feature of living things and under this concept a living human being, like other living organisms, dies when there is an irreversible cessation of the flow of these fluids. The irreversible cessation of heart and lung activity represents a straightforward set of criteria derived from this concept (at least for some animals). Some patients may lose control permanently of their lung function and require ventilation by mechanical means; such patients would still be regarded as alive by all concerned assuming that there was nothing else wrong with them in addition to the problem with the lungs. Even in the event of heart failure and the substitution of the organic heart by an artificial one, the status of such a patient would not change from alive to dead, again assuming that nothing else had changed.

This concept would certainly allow for the formulation of criteria and tests for death. For example, the criteria of death in the human being would be the permanent cessation of heart and lung function and the tests being the appropriate ones for those functions. However, I will argue later that while this flow of vital fluids is a characteristic of living entities, it is merely a manifestation of a complex collection of organic systems and subsystems and that the flow is normally controlled within narrow limits by these systems. I will argue that it is not the flow *per se* but the correctly controlled flow that is important; the full significance of this will be explored later. If there is flow of vital fluids in a living entity, then the flow must be sufficient to keep that entity alive. Since an entity may vary its requirements for energy (for example), the flow of vital fluids must be adjusted appropriately; this adjustment of the flow of vital fluids to match the needs of the entity indicates that some form of control of the flow of vital fluids is necessary. If there is no control of the flow of vital fluids, then at some time the flow of vital fluids will be insufficient for the continued existence of the entity concerned. Hence, whilst the irreversible loss of flow of vital fluids is important and ensures the irreversible loss of control of the flow of vital fluids, it is the control of the flow of vital fluids that is of greater importance.

The Irreversible Loss of the Capacity for Bodily Integration

In general, importance is not placed on the death of a single cell or small group of cells in a large, multi-cellular animal; we are interested in, and place importance on, the death of the entity as a whole. However, a "person as a whole" is not merely a collection of vital fluids in motion but an integrated whole (I have alluded to this in the previous paragraph). Tomlinson has argued that this integrated whole is the essential feature of human life and has suggested that the body's capacity for integrating its functions is the essentially significant indication of life, although he differs from all other authors supporting this monograph by asserting that the normally functioning brain is merely contingent to this integration, *i.e.* its loss is sufficient for but not necessary for the loss of the integration (Tomlinson, 1984).

Veatch argues that this concept has two aspects, and this division seems to meet with widespread agreement (Veatch, 1989a). In this division, the term "bodily integration" has been split into "the integration of the internal bodily environment" and "the integration of one's self with the social environment". According to this view, loss of both of these capacities constitutes death. In view of what comes later in this chapter under the discussion of another concept of death, it is worth stressing at this point that in this concept of death both of these capacities must be lost before the entity that formerly possessed them would be considered to be dead (although Veatch's view seems to be that the loss of the social manifestation is sufficient on its own for death).

If we examine this "two arm" concept in relation to the criteria discussed at the beginning of this document, we find that the first "arm", that is the biological one, could easily apply to all living entities. However, the second "arm", the non-biological or "social" one, poses a problem. In order that an entity demonstrate in its normal state that it has the capacity for integration with the social environment, the entity concerned must possess the property of consciousness. This requirement means that all plants and some animals are excluded from consideration under this concept of death. Much more importantly, however, some human beings are also excluded since there are groups of human beings that do not demonstrate consciousness, namely anencephalic new-borns, those with severe mental retardation and those in irreversible coma. It is my opinion this inability to encompass all human beings is a fatal flaw in this concept of death.

However, this is not the only problem with this second "social" arm of this concept of death. Even if we were to accept that there were some argument that allowed these three groups of human beings, namely anencephalic newborns, those with severe mental retardation and those in irreversible coma, to be included in the "social" arm of this concept (as distinct from exclusion as I have discussed in the preceding paragraph) thereby conceding that this concept of death could encompass all human beings, there would still be problems of the definition of "the integration of oneself with the social environment" and of how to derive criteria and tests for death from it. These problems are not significantly different from the problems encountered with the next concept of death, and it is probably better to discuss them together.

The Irreversible Loss of the Capacity for Consciousness and Social Interaction

This fourth major alternative for a concept of death draws on some of the characteristics of the previous third concept and has often been confused with it. Beecher in 1970 offered a summary of what he thought to be essential to man "his conscious life, his uniqueness, his capacity for remembering, judging, reasoning, acting, enjoying, worrying and so on" (Beecher, 1970). What is remarkable about this list is that it is composed of functions related to or dependent upon consciousness. None of the functions that compose the individual's ability to maintain the internal bodily environment are mentioned.

There is, therefore, a fourth possible concept of death, namely the irreversible loss of the capacity for mental or social functioning. If a human being had lost the capacity for consciousness/mental/social functioning, then they would have lost the essential character of humanness and, according to this concept of death, they would be dead even if they had retained the capacity for integration of their internal environment.

Within this rather broad term "mental or social functioning" there exists a plethora of functions considered by some authors to be ultimately significant to human life. It is worth discussing these separately.

Rationality. It is argued that the human capacity for reasoning is so unique and important that it is the critical, essential feature of human nature. There is some confusion here in that some authors hold the view that some human beings are "persons", namely those who can take part in moral discussion (Englehardt, 1986a; Green and Wickler, 1980; Tooley, 1972; Warren, 1973). For these authors, and others not mentioned, a person is a rights-bearing human being by definition if that human being can take part in moral discussion, while some other human beings are not persons because they are unable to take part in such discussion. I follow the position taken by Veatch (1989b) that the term "person" is synonymous with "living human being" and this is in close agreement with the use of the term in everyday speech by non-philosophers. This position greatly simplifies further discussion and helps to prevent "slippage" or elision from one meaning of the term "person" to another, perhaps more specialised, meaning both in this section and later. With regard to the function of rationality, any concept of death employing this function as a discriminator would be excessively restrictive. By this I mean that the use of the term in this context would not allow the concept of death to encompass all human beings. If one considers the newborn, infants, the severely psychotic or those with severe dementia, the only conclusion one can reach is that no member of these groups of human beings has a capacity for rationality and yet are considered to be alive by all and, indeed, are entitled to certain rights under the law. If one wishes to bring these groups of human beings into the concept of death under discussion, then a function other than rationality needs to be considered.

Consciousness. The use of consciousness as a discriminator between life and death has been argued forcefully by Gervais (1986a). This function would certainly encompass the groups of human beings excluded by the function of rationality, that is use of this function in a concept of death would allow those human beings who are infants or who suffer from severe psychosis or dementia to be considered as alive as, indeed, they are at the present time. However, even this relatively "wide" function ("wide" as opposed to the function of rationality that I consider to be too "narrow") when used in a concept of death poses problems. Let me consider those human beings that are irreversibly unconscious, namely those in the persistent vegetative state (PVS) from whatever cause and those unfortunate to be born anencephalic. In both of these examples, there is no chance of the individuals ever regaining consciousness (one by definition and the other because of total lack of required neurological substrate), yet in both cases I (and I suspect most observers) could not consider them dead, although the anencephalic could be considered as dying. What we have, then, is a group of human beings who are generally considered to be alive and who would be defined as dead under this concept of death if this function of unconsciousness was adopted as the discriminator. Anencephalic infants pose a further problem for this function. I have already mentioned the problem of permanent unconsciousness but I would also like to raise another, related question. The examples of human beings with permanent unconsciousness that I have chosen, *viz.* PVS and anencephaly, differ in one important respect; while a human being who becomes permanently unconscious for some reason (the precise reason is not relevant) has been, at some earlier time, conscious, this is not the case with the anencephalic. These unfortunate individuals lack the necessary anatomical substrate for consciousness (the neocortex) and have never been conscious. This fact of never having been conscious is the important difference between anencephalics and those in PVS. While there may be some form of argument that would allow those in PVS (who had previously been conscious) to be encompassed by a concept of death using consciousness as a discriminator, this argument would not apply to those who had never been conscious. It would seem, therefore, that this discriminator (that is, consciousness) like the function of rationality excludes some human beings from consideration. I have, therefore, to dismiss the function of unconsciousness as a function to be used in any concept of death since it cannot satisfy the most basic of my criteria, namely that it should be able to include all human beings.

Personal identity. This possible function has been proposed by Green and Wickler (1980) and was considered by the President's Commission (1981). They argue that an individual is appropriately considered dead when personal identity (that is, psychological continuity and connectedness) is destroyed. Against this argument I would offer the same group of human beings as before, namely anencephalics, infants, the severely psychotic and those with dementia. No member of this group demonstrates any psychological connectedness or continuity or, at least, none can be demonstrated. I would accept that, in criticism of my argument, there may be an argument that infants have the potential for psychological connectedness and continuity and should be treated accordingly. Even if this criticism were accepted as valid, it does not of course invalidate my argument for anencephalics, the severely psychotic or those with dementia. Veatch offers a test case that is probably more persuasive in rejecting Green and Wickler's suggested function (Veatch, 1989c). This test case involves a subject who develops permanent amnesia and who must build a new life; this subject has a total and irreversible break in psychological continuity and connectedness. The question Veatch asks is "Has the pre-morbid individual died?" Green and Wickler must say that the pre-morbid individual has died and that a new one has been created. That statement, *per se*, is probably acceptable if one interprets the term "dead" in the metaphorical sense. However, Green and Wickler intend that we take the term "dead" in the literal sense and I think that, with that interpretation in mind, Veatch's question about whether or not any appropriate death behaviour should be initiated by society is pertinent. Should this individual's will be enacted, for example? Like Veatch, I (and I suspect the majority of people) think that such death behaviour is entirely inappropriate and should not be initiated; the pre-morbid personality is "dead" but the pre-morbid (physical) person is not. If it is being maintained that the pre-morbid person is dead in the literal sense of the term "dead", then the loss of personal identity is being confused with death as the latter term is generally understood.

Social interaction. It has been a long-held tradition in western culture that a human being is essentially a social animal. However, the claim that the irreversible loss of the capacity for social interaction is to be considered as death is a radical one. It is one that Veatch favours (Veatch, 1989c). To exhibit social interaction (or to have the capacity to do so) at the level discussed by Veatch (1989d) it is necessary for the entity under discussion to have the property of consciousness. My argument against the use of social interaction as a function in any concept of death is, therefore, essentially the same as my argument against the use of consciousness in the same context, that is that there are human beings who cannot be encompassed within the concept of death if the function is used as a discriminator. Whilst Veatch considers in some depth the methods whereby the loss of capacity for consciousness (Veatch, 1989e) may be measured and the criteria applied, such a discussion is rendered irrelevant if one argues, as I do, that to employ the permanent loss of consciousness or the permanent loss of the capacity for social interaction as a criterion of death is a conceptual error. The permanent loss of consciousness or the capacity for social interaction may render a human being less interesting in a moral sense, but it does not classify such a human being as dead (Stanley, 1987; Gillet, 1987).

General Criticism of Those who Support a "Higher Function" or Neocortical Concept of Death

Those who, like myself, accept an organismic concept of human death believe that death is a univocal term. For example, when arguing in favour of an organismic concept of human death, Lamb claims that "the death of a man is no different from that of a dog or a cat" (Lamb, 1985). Gervais rejects this view and argues that "death" can be used equivocally. Gervais believes that human death differs from the death of all other living entities, in that human death has great significance for human relationships and unravels a complex arrangement of rights and responsibilities. She argues:

> "We must make an ethical decision about how best to regard the human for the purposes of declaring death. The death of a person unravels and reconstitutes a complex net of rights and obligations that usually involve many other people.... . We must think of human death not in terms of what it has in common with canine death or feline death, but in terms of what it represents for human relationships: abandonment of all rôles, the end of all interactions, and the reconstituting of rights and obligations. Permanent unconsciousness, whatever its basis, represents these changes." (Gervais, 1986b)

Gervais never denies that it is possible to interpret human death organismically and to take death to have the same meaning for all living organisms. However, she believes that it would be wrong to pursue such a course. In order to accurately represent these differences, Gervais believes that we should declare human beings dead when they cease to exist as persons, that is when they suffer a permanent loss of consciousness. Gervais' position requires that the term "death" be used equivocally for she intends that the term "death" means "irreversible loss of integrated organismic functioning" when referring to non-human entities and "cessation of personal experience" or "permanent loss of consciousness" when referring to human beings.

If we leave to one side the question of whether a non-human animal can have a "complex net of rights and obligations", there is a major problem with Gervais' argument for interpreting "death" equivocally.

Before I discuss this problem in depth, it should be noted that although I am using Gervais' arguments here, similar arguments are put forward by all those who propose a "higher functions" or "neocortical death" concept of death, for example Veatch (1989a), Beecher (1970), Pucetti (1988), Walton (1983), and my arguments against Gervais should be taken as general arguments against this group. The major problem with Gervais' argument is that she assumes that it is possible to use the term "death" in more than one sense. However, unless we want to disregard distinctions that are long established in ordinary language, we must use the term "death" univocally when we speak of the death of any living thing. This univocal use of the term "death" under these circumstances should not be taken to mean that I am implying that the term "death" has only one proper use. The term "death" may have more than one use, for we often make reference to non-living things as "dead", for example "the music died". In this latter sense the term "death" is being used equivocally and in a metaphorical way. However, when we use the term "dead" with reference to living entities, the use of the term must be univocal. Proponents of an organismic concept of life assume that the term "death" is defined as "the loss of life" and they then attempt to make the term "the loss of life" more specific by taking it to mean "the irreversible loss of integrated organismic functioning". Gervais accepts this as one proper use of the term "death" but argues that when the term "death" is applied to human beings the term should be defined as "cessation of one's existence as a person". In this second use, the term "death" is not taken to mean "loss of life" but rather "cessation of existence". However, there is a clear-cut distinction between dying and ceasing to exist. Inanimate objects can cease to exist but cannot properly be said to die. In essence, ordinary language does not identify the term "death" with "cessation of existence" when used in reference to living organisms, although it may when the term "death" is used with reference to non-living things. What the group of "neocortical death" supporters are doing is using the term "death" equivocally and inappropriately.

There is yet another conceptual error that this group has made in arguing for a neocortical concept of death (whatever the precise facet of consciousness that particularly interests them individually). The entire group makes statements of the type "death of the person" when a particular feature of a human being has been permanently lost. What I take to be the meaning of this statement is that the individual concerned has lost some feature of his existence and has, as a consequence of this particular loss, ceased to be a person in the terms that that particular philosopher has defined the term "person". My understanding of this process is that the individual no longer satisfies the particular requirements of the definition of the term "person" but this does not seem, to me at least, to say anything about whether or not that individual's life continues. It seems to me that what is being said when the term "death of a person" is being used by this group of people, is that a particular feature of significant moral value of a human being has been lost and that this loss now excludes the individual from that group of individuals referred to as "persons". Therefore, the question that this group has answered with the phrase "death of a person" is "When does this individual lose that feature that we consider so morally important that the loss of that feature excludes the individual from the group of individuals referred to as persons?". This is the question being answered when Gervais argues that permanent loss of consciousness leads to death of the person (Gervais, 1986b), when Beecher makes the same claim (Beecher, 1970), and when Veatch proposes that permanent loss of social interaction leads to death of the person (Veatch, 1989c). This separation of what is meant by the term "person" and the term "human being" is argued very well by Englehardt (1986b) when he says "not all humans are persons" and

> "The very world of morality is sustained by persons. The problem is that not all humans are persons. ... Infants are not persons. The severely senile and the very severely or profoundly mentally retarded are not persons... Nor are those who are severely brain damaged." (Englehardt, 1986c)

It seems from what has been written by this group of people that they view the term "person" as referring to a human being (leaving aside the question of extraterrestrial life satisfying the requirements for inclusion in the group of individuals covered by the term "person") who has special features, each feature being defined differently by each individual in this group of philosophers. This can be summarised as "person = human being + X", where X is the special feature favoured by a particular philosopher. What has been done after that is that this first question concerning the loss of the morally valuable feature has been conflated with a second question "When does this individual die?" and the answer to the first question has been extended and applied to the second question with the result that we get statements of the type "This human being has lost a particular feature that has moral value and is to be considered to be dead, as a direct consequence of the loss of this particular feature". Two, not totally unconnected, events have happened here. The first is that the term "person" has been defined differently from the meaning that it has in normal speech where it is generally taken to mean "human being" and, under these circumstances, it (that is, the term "person") should be described as being dead only in an equivocal sense of the term "death". However, it is clear that all the philosophers in this group intend that the term "death" used in relation to their own particular definition of the term "person" should be taken in a univocal sense. This use and intended meaning of the term "death" is a fundamental error by all those in this group. The second event is the extension of the answer to the first question, "When does this individual lose that feature that we consider so morally important that the loss of that feature excludes the individual from the group of individuals referred to as persons?" to the second question "When is this individual dead?". These two fundamental errors have been used in the arguments included, in one form or another, by all those who wish to argue for a concept of death that is based upon the loss of "higher functions" or neocortical function.

The controversies concerning definitions of death arise largely from uncertainties surrounding the kind of life that is being declared at an end. As Engelhardt says, "it is one thing to be interested in when human biological life ceases and another to be interested in when persons cease to exist" (Englehardt, 1986d). In this matter of the distinction between biological life and personal or mental life, there is little doubt that the distinction that Engelhardt draws is a real and significant one, but his assertion that concepts of death that do not depend solely upon the function of the neocortex represent a reaction against the conceptual developments that underlie the brain-oriented definition of death is not sustainable. Engelhardt's vision of brain-centred concepts of death is that they can only be used to determine the end of personal life and that the development from a whole-body-oriented concept of death to a whole-brain-oriented concept of death can be interpreted as a move away from a concept of death based on human biological life to a concept of death based on the life of a person (Englehardt, 1986d). However, the concept of death that I advocate in this monograph is, most definitely, a brain-centred concept of death and yet is based upon the assumption that it is the biological life of an individual that is important, not the loss of certain features contingent upon the presence of life, when death of the individual is to be determined.

Summary

In this section, I have argued against the current concepts of death. The earlier concepts of death, namely the irreversible loss of the soul from the body and the irreversible cessation of flow of vital fluids appear to me to be insupportable. The capacity for bodily integration is more promising but the weakness is in the second "arm" of the concept; a similar weakness exists in the concepts of death that employ the "higher functions" of rationality, consciousness, personal identity and social interaction. This weakness is not, as some would argue, in the difficulty of measuring these criteria but resides more basically in the fact that these criteria would exclude from consideration some groups of human beings. It is my contention that, at a minimum, any concept of death should be able to encompass all human beings.

References

Beecher, H.K. (1970), *The new definition of death, some opposing views*. Unpublished paper presented at the meeting of the American Association for the Advancement of Science, Dec. 1970. (Quoted in Tomlinson, T. (1984), "The conservative use of the brain death criteria: a critique", *J. Med. and Philosophy*, vol. 9(4), pp. 377-393). See also, Beecher, H.K. (1969), "After the 'definition of irreversible coma'", *New Eng. J. Med.*, vol. 281, p. 1070.

Browne, A. (1983), "Whole brain death reconsidered", *J. Med. Ethics*, vol. 9, pp. 28-31.

Englehardt, H.T. Jr. (1986a), *The foundations of bioethics*, Oxford Univ. Press, New York, pp. 104-127.

Englehardt, H.T. Jr. (1986b), *The foundations of bioethics*, Oxford Univ. Press, New York, p. 108.

Englehardt, H.T. Jr. (1986c), *The foundations of bioethics*, Oxford Univ. Press, New York, p. 202.

Englehardt, H.T. Jr. (1986d), *The foundations of bioethics*, Oxford Univ. Press, New York, p. 204.

Gervais, K.G. (1986a), *Redefining death*, Yale Univ. Press, New Haven, pp. 159-182.

Gervais, K.G. (1986b), *Redefining death*, Yale Univ. Press, New Haven, p.152.

Gillett, G. (1987), "Reply to JM Stanley: fiddling and clarity", *J. Med. Ethics*, vol. 13(1), pp. 23-25.

Green, M.B. and Wickler, D. (1980), "Brain death and personal identity", *Philosophy and Public Affairs*, vol. 9(2), pp. 105-133.

Lamb, D. (1985a), *Death, brain death and ethics*, Croom Helm, London, p. 12.

Lamb, D. (1985b), *Death, brain death and ethics*, Croom Helm, London, p. 7.

Pallis, C. (1983a), "Whole brain death reconsidered: physiological facts and philosophy", *J. Med. Ethics*, vol. 9, pp. 32-37.

Pallis, C. (1983b), *ABC of brain stem death*, British Medical Assoc., London, p. 2.

Pope Pius XII (1957), "Prolongation of life", *Pope Speaks*, vol. 4, pp. 393-398.

President's Commission for the study of ethical problems in medicine and biomedical and behavioural research; medical, legal and ethical issues in the definition of death (1981), US Government Printing Office, Washington DC, pp. 39-40.

Pucetti, R. (1988), "Does anyone survive neocortical death?", in R.M. Zaner (ed.), *Death: beyond whole brain criteria* : Kluwer Academic, Boston, pp. 75-90.

Stanley, J.M. (1987), "More fiddling with the definition of death?", *J. Med. Ethics*, vol. 13(1), pp. 21-22.

Tomlinson, T. (1984), "The conservative use of the brain death criteria: a critique", *J. Med. and Philosophy*, vol. 9(4), pp. 377-393.

Tooley, M. (1972), "Abortion and infanticide", *Philosophy and Public Affairs*, vol. 2, pp. 37-65.

Veatch, R. M. (1989a), *Death, dying and the biological revolution*, Yale Univ. Press, New Haven, pp. 19-32.

Veatch, R.M. (1989b), *Death, dying and the biological revolution*, Yale Univ. Press, New Haven, pp. 26-27.

Veatch, R.M. (1989c), *Death, dying and the biological revolution*, Yale Univ. Press, New Haven, p. 28.

Veatch, R.M. (1989d), *Death, dying and the biological revolution*, Yale Univ. Press, New Haven, pp. 28-29.

Veatch, R.M. (1989e), *Death, dying and the biological revolution*, Yale Univ. Press, New Haven, pp. 39-41.

Walton, D.N. (1983), *Ethics of withdrawal of life support systems*, Praeger, New York, (reprinted 1987, version referred to), p. 82.

Warren, M.A. (1973), "On the moral and legal status of abortion", *The Monist*, vol. 57, pp. 43-61.

5 Consideration of Different Brain States in Relation to Different Concepts of Death

"I go whence I shall not return, even to the land of darkness and the shadow of death"
Job ch. 10, v. 20

Introduction

I have previously discussed at some length and in some detail the existence of a variety of altered brain states and the clinical manifestation of these states (see chapter 3). I did not, at that time, discuss those different brain states in terms of the different concepts of death that have been advocated and I will now turn my attention to that. I shall not necessarily discuss them in the same order as before simply because the relative importance of each state is not necessarily the same in this discussion as it was in the earlier chapter.

Brain Death

As a term for an altered brain state for discussion in this section, this term has little to commend it—I have already alluded to the confusion that may arise with its use. I intend, therefore to discuss "brain death" under more precise headings.

Whole Brain Death

This term is self-explanatory and is a state in which all functions of the brain including cortical, subcortical and brainstem functions are permanently lost. It should be remembered that this does not mean that all cells in the brain are dead, but rather that the functions of the brain have been permanently lost. This altered brain state is one state that satisfies the criteria of all of the concepts of death previously discussed except the position taken by Jonas (1974), Evans (1990), Truog (1997) and Shewmon

(1997). With the exception of these four philosophers, all other commentators referred to here would view a human being with whole brain death as dead. Some, however, would view whole brain death as being unnecessarily conservative. Veatch (1975, 1989a) considers that "death means a complete change in the status of a living entity characterised by the irreversible loss of those characteristics that are essentially significant to it" and that "these characteristics" are contained in the capacity for social interaction. The requirement of the loss of the capacity for social interaction does not necessarily require whole brain death for its fulfilment but only the death of a much smaller area of the brain, the neocortex. Gervais (1986) argues that the permanent loss of consciousness constitutes death of the person; such permanent loss of consciousness whilst occurring in whole brain death is also a feature of both brainstem death and neocortical death and, therefore, does not require whole brain death as a criterion. Gervais argues strongly that neocortical death is sufficient for the diagnosis of death of the person and that whole brain death is unnecessarily conservative, a stance that is shared with Veatch.

Pucetti (1988) argues that the capacity for personal experience is of ultimate concern to us morally and that it would be irrational to hold the view that any person who has sustained permanent loss of consciousness is alive; in his analogy, he specifically cites neocortical death as the criterion required for the permanent loss of consciousness. However, Walton (1983a) whilst accepting that the permanent loss of consciousness constitutes death of the person and that neocortical death would produce permanent loss of consciousness, argues that the present state of medical knowledge concerning brain function and recovery does not allow of sufficient certainty in the diagnosis of neocortical death. For this reason, he argues that the adoption of whole brain death as the death of the person is to be preferred, since it is more secure. Finally, Smith (1988) has argued that the law (at least in the USA) should consider neocortical death as defining the death of the person.

Brainstem Death

If we accept that the term "whole brain death" describes a state in which all functions of the brain have been permanently lost, then by analogy the term "brainstem death" should describe a state in which all functions of the brainstem have been permanently lost. This conclusion is not, however, substantiated by empirical observation. I have already discussed in chapter 2 that Wetzel *et al* (1985) described a series of brain dead patients in all of whom changes in blood pressure similar to those seen in non-brainstem dead patients were evoked by surgical incision in the case of organ removal. The authors concluded that these responses were probably attributable to some residual brainstem function. They emphasised that the current (in this case, 1985) criteria for the diagnosis of brainstem death were not intended "to identify total cessation of function of all brainstem neurones". Another report (Aitkenhead and Thomas, 1987) demonstrated the persistence of function of some of the brainstem nuclei of brainstem dead patients, in terms of muscular activity in the lower part of the oesophagus. Spontaneous oesophageal muscular contraction is believed to be dependent upon activity of the brainstem. Another clinician (Sinclair, 1987) offered two possible explanations for this observation of retained function of brainstem nuclei in brainstem dead patients. The first explanation was that spontaneous lower oesophageal muscular contraction was an intrinsic response of the oesophagus "for which there is no evidence, all the evidence pointing in the opposite direction". The other explanation invoked "some residual function in the oesophageal motility centre (in the brainstem) for which the current clinical tests are insufficiently sensitive". Another report on the same subject, that is the persistence of spontaneous oesophageal muscular contraction in patients diagnosed as brainstem dead, concluded that "the brainstem activity reported may not represent life in all its fullness, but neither does it equate with death" (Hill, 1987). It seems from these reports that the term "brainstem death" could not reasonably be taken to mean the permanent loss of all functions of the brainstem. In addition to the residual functions of the brainstem present at the diagnosis of brainstem death, there is also evidence that the pituitary gland continues to function at the time of the diagnosis of brainstem death, indicating that brainstem death does not necessarily imply death of other areas of the brain (Fackler and Rogers, 1987; Hall, Mashiter, Lumley and Robson, 1980; Schrader, Krogness, Aakvaag, Sortland and Purvis, 1980; Robertson, Hramiak and Gelb, 1989). It is possible, then, that control of homeostasis persists for some time after brainstem death if ventilation of the patient continues. Eventually, however, all the oesophageal muscular activity, the haemodynamic responses and the hypothalamic-pituitary function cease. Brainstem death has then resulted in whole brain death for all practical purposes.

  Brainstem death (with or without the responses discussed above) would be viewed as death by Pallis (1983), Beecher (1969), Lamb (1985a), Gervais (1986) and Veatch (1975, 1989a) although for slightly different reasons; the basic underlying reason is that there is permanent unconsciousness coupled with a permanent loss of breathing although for the latter two the absence or presence of breathing has no role in the determination of the ontological status of an individual. Any concept of death that has permanent loss of consciousness as a sole criterion or that has another criterion that is dependent upon the presence of consciousness (for example the "social interaction" criterion of Veatch) would have the criterion satisfied by brainstem death. However, let me consider the term "brainstem death". As I have discussed earlier in this chapter and also in chapter 2, this term cannot be taken to mean the permanent loss of all brainstem functions. However, there are other possible interpretations of the term "brainstem death":

- Permanent loss of some if not all of the functions of the brainstem alone. This I will refer to as the "narrow" definition of brainstem death.
- Permanent loss of the functions of the brainstem and, in addition, the permanent loss of function of other areas of the brain occurring as a consequence of brainstem death. This will be referred to as the "broad" definition of brainstem death.

The "narrow" definition of brainstem death would seem to be the definition that is arrived at by common-sense usage of the words in the term "brainstem death" and there is no doubt that this "narrow" definition would satisfy the various criteria of death advocated by Veatch (1975, 1989a), Gervais (1986), Pallis (1983) and Beecher (1969). If we accept, for the moment, the narrow definition of brainstem death, that is the one in which the rest of the brain is working, then using the concept of death that I am advocating a human being in this state would be considered to be alive since homeostasis would be expected to be maintained.

However, this narrow definition of brainstem death is one that exists only in intellectual or philosophical discussion and, in practice, there is permanent loss of function of the remainder of the brain at about the same time as brainstem death occurs, that is the "broad" definition of brainstem death applies. This means that, in practice, the state referred to as brainstem death is for all practical purposes the state of whole brain death. The result of this is that, again, all the suggested concepts of death (including my own) would view this state as death; the exceptions are, as before, Jonas (1974), Evans (1990), Truog (1997) and Shewmon (1997).

Neocortical Death

As I have previously explained in chapter 3, this term refers to the death of the cerebral cortex, and results in permanent loss of consciousness but with an intact ability to breathe and to maintain homeostasis. It follows from this permanent loss of consciousness that any advocate of a concept of death that has this as a criterion or of a concept of death that has another criterion that depends upon consciousness being present, will view the state of neocortical death as death of a human being. This group of advocates will include Beecher (1969), Gervais (1986) and Veatch (1975, 1989a). Others such as Pallis (1983), myself and the conservative Jonas (1974), Evans (1990), Truog (1997) and Shewmon (1997) whose concepts of death neither include permanent unconsciousness as a sole criterion nor include it at all as a criterion will, consequently, view anyone with neocortical death as being alive. The clinical correlate of neocortical death, as I have mentioned already in chapter 3, is most commonly referred to as the persistent vegetative state. This differs significantly from whole brain death (or brainstem death as discussed in the preceding paragraphs) in that the human being in the persistent vegetative state will continue to maintain bodily integrity if supplied with the normal requirements for this, namely food and drink, whereas a human being who is in the state of brain death cannot maintain bodily integrity. Recent attempts to try to maintain human beings from this latter group in as normal a physiological state as possible have met with no success. A published description of such an attempt at "maintenance" is that described by Singer (1995a). The essential facts of this case are that an 18-year-old woman who was 13 weeks pregnant was declared brain dead after a road traffic accident. Attempts were made to maintain the woman's body in as near a normal physiological state as possible but this failed and a spontaneous abortion followed approximately 5 weeks after the accident. This should be contrasted with the case of Elaine Esposito (described by Walton (1983b)) who is the longest recorded survivor in the persistent vegetative state. She survived in this condition for 37 years 3 months and 37 days after developing ischaemic brain damage at age 6 years.

This clinical state (that is, the persistent vegetative state) is the state that most commonly produces ethical dilemmas for those who wish to argue for or against euthanasia, but that is a separate issue that will not be discussed further although it should be noted that anyone involved in either side in this debate has already conceded that the persistent vegetative state is a state in which a person is considered to be alive, since there would be little point in discussing euthanasia if the state was one in which the patients were considered to be dead. A recent, well-publicised case of persistent vegetative state or neocortical death was that of Tony Bland. In 1989, this 17 year old boy was involved in the worst disaster in British sporting history (Hillsborough disaster) and sustained extensive and permanent damage to his neocortex as a result of prolonged hypoxia. A good report of the pertinent details of this case has been published by Singer (1995b). There was no doubt medically that Tony Bland was in the persistent vegetative state and I quote from Singer (who, in turn, is quoting Lord Justice Hoffmann (1993)):

> "Since April 15 1989 Tony Bland has been in persistent vegetative state. He lies in Airedale General Hospital in Keighley, fed liquid food by a pump through a tube passing through his nose and down the back of his throat into the stomach. His bladder is emptied through a catheter inserted through his penis, which from time to time has caused infections requiring dressing and antibiotic treatment. His stiffened joints have caused his limbs to be rigidly contracted so that his arms are tightly flexed across his chest and his legs unnaturally contorted. Reflex movements in the throat cause him to vomit and dribble. Of all this, and the presence of family members who take turns to visit him, Anthony Bland has no consciousness at all. The parts of his brain, which provided him with consciousness, have turned to fluid. The darkness and oblivion, which descended at Hillsborough, will never depart. His body is alive, but he has no life in the sense that even the most pitifully handicapped but conscious human being has a life. But the advances of modern medicine permit him to be kept in this state for years, even perhaps for decades."

Despite the physical changes in Tony Bland, Singer does not seem to be in any doubt that his body is alive although "he has no life in the sense that even the most pitifully handicapped but conscious human being has life" (Singer, 1995c).

This, then, is the state that Beecher (1969), Veatch (1975, 1989a), Gervais (1986) and Pucetti (1988) would argue constitutes death and the state that Smith (1988) advocates we view as death for legal purposes. On the other hand, the position taken by Singer (1995b) that human beings in this state are alive but have no obvious quality of life is one that is also adopted by Pallis (1983), Lamb (1985a), Jonas (1974), Evans (1990), Truog (1997), Shewmon (1997) and myself.

Locked-in Syndrome

A human being in this state demonstrates consciousness albeit by means of an extremely limited means of communication, namely eye movement and blinking, and there is a limited ability to maintain bodily integrity in that spontaneous breathing cannot occur and artificial ventilation is required. A human being in this condition demonstrates consciousness and all other attributes that depend upon the presence of consciousness, for example social interaction, although this demonstration is limited as a result of the physical disabilities contingent upon the condition. There is no doubt, once communication has been established with a human being in this condition, that such a human being is awake, aware and in control of normal "higher brain" functions such as abstract thought. There is no doubt that such a human being is considered to be alive under all currently accepted or suggested concepts of death. The state of the locked-in syndrome, while rare (I have personal experience of only two cases) and of great interest to neurologists, does not seem to pose a problem to philosophers in terms of ontological status. A recent article has illustrated this very well (Herbert, 1997). The editor of Elle magazine suffered a stroke and was considered to be a "vegetable" with control over only his left eye-lid. He was diagnosed as being in the locked-in syndrome but he has recently published a book after learning to communicate by means of blinking his left eye-lid. A better illustration of the retention of the "higher" mental functions in the locked-in syndrome despite the appalling physical limitations can hardly be imagined.

It would be instructive, at this point, to compare the locked-in syndrome with the previously discussed state of brainstem death. The locked-in syndrome is a result of permanent loss of function of part of the brainstem and I have already argued that brainstem death is permanent loss of function of the brainstem but not of all the functions of the brainstem. Both brainstem death and the locked-in syndrome can, therefore, be described as being the result of permanent loss of some of the functions of the brainstem; the essential difference between them is that in the locked-in syndrome the Reticular Activating System (RAS) is intact and consciousness is retained, whereas in brainstem death the function of the RAS has been permanently lost and consciousness has been permanently lost as a direct consequence. The only difference between the locked-in syndrome and brainstem death is the loss of function of the RAS and the consequent permanent loss of consciousness. It would also be interesting to speculate here about the responses by the advocates of the currently accepted and proposed concepts of death on a condition in which the function of the RAS had been permanently lost but in which the other functions of the brainstem are intact. This would result in a permanently unconscious human being but with spontaneous breathing and control of homeostasis. Since this description matches the description of the persistent vegetative state albeit from a different pathology, I have no doubt that Beecher (1969), Veatch (1975, 1989a), and Gervais (1986) would consider such a human being as dead. Others such as Pallis (1983), Lamb (1985a), Jonas (1974), Evans (1990), Pucetti (1988), Singer (1995a), Truog (1997), Shewmon (1997) and myself would consider such a human being to be alive for a variety of reasons, for example because of intact breathing (Pallis), spontaneous breathing and heartbeat (Jonas, Evans), intact integration (Lamb) and intact homeostasis (myself).

Akinetic Mutism

While a human being in this state demonstrates consciousness, the lack of evidence of any mental activity in this state produces problems for those who hold that any concept of death should include functions that depend on the presence of consciousness, for example Veatch (1975, 1989a), Gervais (1986) and Beecher (1969). The problem with this condition for those who advocate a "neocortical death" concept of death is that a human being in this condition exhibits alertness but does not exhibit any evidence of other mental activity. If we are to accept that consciousness is the all-important criterion for the determination of the ontological status of a human being in terms of death, as advocated by Beecher (1969), Gervais (1986), Pucetti (1988) and Cranford and Smith (1979) then any individual with akinetic mutism is to be viewed unequivocally as alive. This ontological status is also the one accorded by Pallis (1983) and Lamb (1985a) because of spontaneous breathing, consciousness and bodily integration, Jonas (1974), Evans (1990), Truog (1997) and Shewmon (1997) because of spontaneous heartbeat and breathing and myself because of the evidence for spontaneous control of homeostasis. However, the status of such individuals is less clear if one considers the concepts of death advocated by Veatch (1975, 1989a) and Green and Wickler (1980). Green and Wickler argue that an individual is appropriately considered dead when personal identity is destroyed; they define personal identity as "psychological continuity and connectedness". In an individual with akinetic mutism there is no evidence of either psychological continuity or connectedness and while I accept that this lack of evidence for these two criteria is not the same as actual lack of the same two criteria, it does raise doubts about how Green and Wickler would classify such an individual. The criteria advocated by Veatch (1989b) for death is the permanent loss of the capacity for social interaction. However, he goes on to say that the capacity for social interaction and the capacity for consciousness are coterminous and that "for all practical purposes it may make no difference whether we speak of the critical characteristic as capacity for consciousness or social interaction". He also states that "even though it is crucial for a philosophical understanding of the human's nature to distinguish between these two functions, it may not be necessary for deciding when an individual has died". Veatch thus sees these two criteria as essentially the same and while he discusses the problems for his concept of death posed by human beings with severe mental handicap, he does not, apparently, foresee the problems posed by the condition of akinetic mutism. The problem for Veatch posed by this condition is that the capacity for consciousness and the capacity for social interaction have been separated and while the human being with akinetic mutism appears to demonstrate consciousness, there is no concomitant demonstration of social interaction. Those human beings with akinetic mutism, therefore, fail to demonstrate the one feature that Veatch considers "is essential for being treated as alive". Would Veatch classify as dead those human beings with akinetic mutism? His answer to this question is to say "for our purposes we can say that the concept of death is one in which the essential element that is lost is the capacity for consciousness or social interaction or both" (Vetach, 1989c), a statement that does not really answer the question. Veatch's stance becomes clearer if one considers his arguments for the measurement of the loss of the criteria for death and the locus of death; in neither case does he discuss the measurement of the loss of social interaction or the locus of such a loss but restricts himself to discussion of the measurement of the loss of the capacity for consciousness and its locus. It would seem that for Veatch the loss of the capacity for consciousness appears to be vital in the determination of death and, accordingly, it would seem likely that he would view a human being with akinetic mutism as being alive.

If the concept of death that I advocate, namely the permanent loss of the control of homeostasis, is examined here we find that there is no disparity between the common-sense view and that concept; in both cases human beings in the state of akinetic mutism are viewed as live as, indeed, they are by Jonas (1974), Evans (1990), Truog (1997) and Shewmon (1997).

Coma

There is little clinical difference between this state and the persistent vegetative state although the latter may have "sleep-wake" cycles. Consequently, much of my argument in the section on the persistent vegetative state is applicable to coma. Advocates of concepts of death that would be satisfied with neocortical death or the persistent vegetative state will also be satisfied with the clinical condition of coma and Beecher (1969), Gervais (1986), Veatch (1975, 1989a), Cranford and Smith (1979) and Pucetti (1988) would hold that permanent coma represents death of the person and that human beings in coma are dead. On the other hand, those whose concepts of death are not satisfied by the permanent loss of consciousness alone such as Jonas (1974), Evans (1990), Pallis (1983), Lamb (1985a), Truog (1997), Shewmon (1997) and myself would view a human being in permanent coma as being alive. The position of Walton (1983a) with regard to coma (and persistent vegetative state) is interesting. His concept of death (permanent loss of consciousness) could and would be satisfied by both the clinical states of persistent vegetative state and permanent coma. However, his argument, using tutioristic reasoning, is that we should "play safe" and he will not accept any clinical state other than whole brain death as satisfying his criteria for death. He must, therefore view a human being in permanent coma as being alive.

Anencephaly

This term, as I have explained in greater depth in an earlier chapter on altered brain states, is applied to new-borns who have been born with the cerebral hemispheres of their brain missing. They are not born as Singer states with "only a brainstem" (Singer, 1995d). Such babies have normal heartbeat, breathing and reflexes but have no consciousness; they can be described as being in a persistent vegetative state (Campbell, 1991). Anencephalic babies usually die within a few hours of birth and only about 1% survive for 3 months or more, but this may merely reflect the lack of effort to keep them alive (Shewmon, 1988); there is one well-documented case of an anencephalic baby surviving for several years (Gianelli, 1994).

Arguments similar to those I put forward in the section on the persistent vegetative state can be used here to show that Gervais (1986) and Veatch (1975, 1989a) would view an anencephalic baby as dead; Beecher's position (1969) would be unclear, as it was before. Advocates of brainstem death such as Pallis (1983) and Lamb (1985b) would view such babies as alive as would Jonas (1974), Evans (1990), Truog (1997) and Shewmon (1997). Walton's (1983a) position would be the same as in coma and the persistent vegetative state in that he would argue for a concept of death that, technically, requires only neocortical death but demands whole brain death as the criterion; he would view anencephalic babies as alive for this reason. The concept of death that I argue for in this monograph allows me to view anencephalic babies as alive.

Summary

What I have done, in this chapter, is to illustrate the various abnormal brain states that I had discussed in clinical and pathological terms in chapter 3 in terms of the present concepts of death. If we exclude, for the moment, the conservative advocates who do not advocate a brain-centred concept of death, it can be seen that there is general agreement in only some of these brain states, namely whole brain death and the locked-in syndrome; any human being in either of these two states would be viewed as dead, in the case of whole brain death, or alive in the case of the locked-in syndrome. It is, perhaps, more interesting to examine the altered brain states upon which there is no general agreement between the various concepts of death. The first of these states is brainstem death. If we examine this in the narrow sense (of brainstem death) that I discussed earlier, we come to the conclusion that a human being who is capable of maintaining bodily integrity (apart from breathing) would be viewed as dead by all those who advocate a brain-centred concept of death except me. The brain-centred concept of death that I put forward in this monograph would allow me to join with the advocates of a conservative, non-brain-centred concept of death in classifying a human being in such a state (namely brainstem death) as alive. What the former group of brain-centred concept of death advocates is doing is asking that a human being should be pronounced dead when any other animal in the same state would be considered to be alive. Whilst accepting that this narrow definition of brainstem death may only exist for a relatively short time (perhaps a few hours at most), I would repeat that the advocates of brainstem death must be prepared to accept this anomaly. The alternative would be for them to accept, in theory, the broad definition of brainstem death which is, in practice, the clinical state of a human being when brainstem death is pronounced in a clinical setting. Whilst they may accept this in practice, accepting it in theory would require them to admit that the term "brainstem death" is actually "whole brain death" both in practice and in theory. It is not clear if any advocate of brainstem death has addressed this dilemma. The potential problem that I touched upon earlier in this section, namely that of two standards of death—one for humans and another for animals—is one that is raised by the brainstem concept of death as I have indicated but is more strongly raised by the concept of neocortical death. I agree with Lamb (1985b) when he says "it does not make sense to speak of one kind of death for humans and another kind for other life forms". I have already argued earlier in this monograph for a uniform concept of death that would be applicable to all animals; such a concept as I suggest and as I have put forward in this monograph would not produce this glaring inconsistency in standards. If we turn our attention to the state of brainstem death as it is practised (see the second paragraph under the heading "Brainstem death"), we find that there is no disagreement between the different brain-centred concepts of death. The reason for this is that the whole brain is dead (although that is not a requirement in brainstem death) when brainstem death is pronounced in the UK in the vast majority of cases and I have already discussed that state in terms of the different concepts (see above).

Any human being in the state of neocortical death would be considered to be alive by an advocate of the brainstem concept of death, by Jonas (1974), Evans (1990), Truog (1997), Shewmon (1997) and by the concept I put forward in this monograph; advocates of all other brain-centred concepts of death (Gervais (1986), Beecher (1969), Veatch (1975, 1989a), Puccetti (1988)) would consider such human beings to be dead. The position of Walton (1983(b)) is unclear since the state of neocortical death would satisfy his theoretical concept of death, it would not satisfy his practical concept of death. My reason for considering humans in the state of neocortical death (or persistent vegetative state) to be alive is essentially the same argument that I put forward for considering those in the brainstem death state (narrow definition) to be alive, that is, the presence of control of homeostasis.

References

Aitkenhead, A.R. and Thomas, D.I. (1987), "Lower oesophageal contractility as an indicator of brain death in paralysed and mechanically ventilated patients with head injury", *Brit. Med. J.*, vol. 294, p. 1287.

Beecher, H.K. (1969), "After the definition of irreversible coma", *New Eng. J. Med.*, vol. 281, pp. 1070-1071.

Campbell, N. (1991), "Some anatomy and physiology", in K. Saunders and B. Moore (eds.), *Anencephalics, infants and brain death: treatment options and the issue of organ donation*, Law Reform Commission of Victoria, Melbourne, p. 13.

Cranford, R.E. and Smith, H.L. (1979), "Some critical distinctions between brain death and persistent vegetative state", *Ethics in Science and Medicine*, vol. 6, pp. 199-209.

Evans, M. (1990), "A plea for the heart", *Bioethics*, vol. 4(3), pp. 227-231.

Fackler, J.C. and Rogers, M.C. (1987), "Is brain death really cessation of all intracranial function?", *J. Paediatrics*, vol. 110, pp. 84-86.

Gervais, K.G. (1986), *Redefining death*. Yale Univ. Press, New Haven, 1986.

Gianelli, D. (1994), "Doctors argue futility of treating anencephalic baby", *American Medical News*, vol. 37(11), p. 5. Also, Greenhouse, L. (1994), "Court order to treat baby with partial brain prompts debate on costs and ethics", *New York Times*, vol. 20 Feb. (Both quoted in Singer, P. (1995), *Rethinking life and death*, Oxford Univ. Press, Oxford.)

Green, M.B. and Wikler, D. (1980), "Brain death and personal identity", *Philosophy and Public Affairs*, vol. 9, pp. 105-133.

Hall, G.M., Mashiter, K., Lumley, J. and Robson, J.G. (1980), "Hypothalamic pituitary function in the 'brain dead' patient", *Lancet*, vol. 2, p. 1259.

Herbert, S. (1997), "Paralysed editor silences chattering classes with a wink", *The Daily Telegraph*, Mar 6, p. 19.

Hill, D.J. (1987), "Lower oesophageal contractility as an indicator of brain death in paralysed and mechanically ventilated patients with head injury", *Brit. Med. J.*, vol. 294, p. 1488.

Hoffmann, L-J. (1993), "Airedale NHS Trust v Bland (CA)", *Weekly Law Reports*, vol. 19 February, p. 350.

Jonas, H. (1974), "Against the stream: comments on the definition and redefinition of death", in H. Jonas, *Philosophical essays: from ancient creed to technological man*, Univ. of Chicago Press, Chicago, (reprinted 1980).

Lamb, D. (1985a), *Death, brain death and ethics*, Croom Helm Ltd, Beckenham.

Lamb, D. (1985b), *Death, brain death and ethics*, Croom Helm Ltd, Beckenham, p. 93.

Pallis, C. (1983), *The ABC of brain stem death*, Brit. Med. Assoc., London.

Pucetti, R. (1988), "Does anyone survive neocortical death?", in R.M. Zaner (ed.), *Beyond whole brain criteria*, Kluwer Academic Publishers, Boston, pp. 75-80.

Robertson, K.M., Hramiak, I.M. and Gelb, A.W. (1989), "Endocrine changes and haemodynamic stability after brain death", *Transplant Proceedings*, vol. 21, pp. 1197-1198.

Schrader, H., Krogness, K., Aakvaag, A., Sortland, O. and Purvis, K. (1980), "Changes of pituitary hormones in brain death", *Acta Neurochirurgica*, vol. 52, pp. 239-248.

Shewmon, D. (1988), "Anencephaly: selected medical aspects", *Hastings Center Report*, vol. 18(5), pp. 11-19.

Shewmon, D.A. (1997), "Recovery from 'brain death': a neurologist's apologia", *Linacre Quarterly*, Feb, p. 30.

Sinclair, M.E. (1987), "Lower oesophageal contractility as an indicator of brain death in paralysed and mechanically ventilated patients with head injury", *Brit. Med. J.*, vol. 294, p. 1488.
Singer, P. (1995a), *Rethinking life and death*, Oxford Univ. Press, Oxford, pp. 12-16.
Singer, P. (1995b), *Rethinking life and death*, Oxford Univ. Press, Oxford, pp. 57-60.
Singer, P. (1995c), *Rethinking life and death*, Oxford Univ. Press, Oxford, p. 58.
Singer, P. (1995d), *Rethinking life and death*, Oxford Univ. Press, Oxford, p. 38.
Smith, D.R. (1988), "Legal issues leading to the notion of neocortical death", in R.M. Zaner (ed.), *Beyond whole brain criteria*, Kluwer Academic Publishers, Boston, pp. 111-144.
Truog, R.D. (1997), "Is it time to abandon brain death?", *Hastings Centre Report*, vol. 27(1), pp. 29-37.
Veatch, R.M. (1975), "The whole brain oriented concept of death: an outmoded philosophical formulation", *J. Thanatology*, vol. 3, pp. 13-30.
Veatch, R.M. (1989a), *Death, dying and the biological revolution*, Yale Univ. Press, New Haven, p. 17.
Veatch, R.M. (1989b), *Death, dying and the biological revolution*, Yale Univ. Press, New Haven, pp. 28 and 293.
Veatch, R.M. (1989c), *Death, dying and the biological revolution*, Yale Univ. Press, New Haven, p. 29.
Walton, D.N. (1983a), *Ethics of withdrawal of life support systems*, Praeger, New York, (reprinted 1987, version referred to), p. 82.
Walton, D.N. (1983b), *Ethics of withdrawal of life support systems*, Praeger, New York, (reprinted 1987, version referred to), p. 79.
Wetzel, R,C., Setzer, N., Stiff, J.L. and Rogers, M.C. (1985), "Haemodynamic responses in brain dead organ donor patients", *Anaesthesia and Analgesia*, vol. 64, pp. 125-128.

6 Can There Be Necessary and Sufficient Conditions for Life?

"As though to breathe were life"
Alfred, Lord Tennyson *Ulysses* 1.6

Introduction

I shall attempt to answer the question about whether or not there can be necessary and sufficient conditions for life by firstly examining the question "What is life?" and thereafter by examining the features that living entities possess. This latter examination will have two approaches. The first approach will be to look at an animal such as a human being and examine what features are necessary for the continuing existence of such an animal. The second approach will be to look at what basic common features exist in all living entities. By using these two approaches, I hope to provide a strong argument that there are, indeed, necessary and sufficient conditions for life. One area that must be discussed here, prior to further discussion, is to distinguish clearly between two possible interpretations of the idea of sufficient conditions for life. What must be distinguished is the difference between:
- the idea of saying, of a particular individual or entity, that there are sufficient conditions for regarding that individual or entity as alive;

and
- the idea of positing, *ab initio*, generally sufficient conditions for life to occur.

The distinction between these two interpretations of the idea of sufficient conditions of life is similar to the distinction between a clinician diagnosing the condition of a patient in terms of whether he or she is alive or dead and a palaeontologist predicting the occurrence of life at some point in pre-history. There would be considerable difficulty in establishing any claim that, given certain conditions, life is bound to occur but this difficulty is of no immediate concern to me; my concern and interest lie not with the latter idea but with the former idea of sufficient conditions for life.

What is Life?

It would seem tautological to say that an entity is living when it possesses the property of life, but it is perhaps easier to explore the meaning of my original question ("Can there be necessary and sufficient conditions for life?") from this approach. I now need to explore and try to answer the question "What is life?" What is being asked when such a question is raised is an enquiry about the characteristic feature of life, that is about the feature or property of an entity that causes us to categorise that entity as being alive. What is it that causes us to say that a lump of matter is alive? (I am not limiting the discussion to human beings at this point.) Schrödinger (1944) put forward a tentative answer to this question in terms that a physicist would understand and only after a discussion of the laws of thermodynamics. I believe that his answer provides a basis for the selection of the ability to maintain homeostasis as the feature of human life that is of primary importance in the assessment of whether or not a human being is dead or alive. I would, therefore, like to explore and expand on the comments by Schrödinger (1944). He begins by suggesting that we would consider something to be alive when it "goes on 'doing something'...for a much longer period than we would expect an inanimate piece of matter to 'keep going' under similar circumstances". He suggests that the "doing something" consists of "moving, exchanging material with its environment, and so forth". Certainly, if a lump of matter that is not alive is isolated or placed in a uniform environment, all motion soon ceases, all electrical and chemical potentials or differences are reduced to zero and the temperature of the lump of matter equals that of the environment. This state is permanent and is referred to by physicists as the state of thermodynamic equilibrium or the state of maximum entropy.

A common feature of all entities considered to be alive is that this state of thermodynamic equilibrium or maximum entropy is avoided, *i.e.* such a state is not found in entities considered to be alive. In order to achieve the avoidance of this state of maximum entropy, the entity must put energy into the system and this energy is obtained from the metabolism of the entity concerned. In other words, a living entity in order to avoid the state of maximum entropy must extract energy from substances in the environment (*e.g.* sunlight, carbohydrates, fats and proteins) and use this energy to control the state of entropy. Prior to discussion of the relevance of this to the main thrust of my argument, it would be pertinent to offer an explanation of what is meant by the term "entropy". Schrödinger expounds on this in some detail in terms and mathematics (1944), as does the CRC

Handbook (1979), but I am not sure that matters are clarified for the non-specialist. For the purposes of this discussion, entropy can be thought of as a measure of chaos or dispersion of energy in a system; low entropy implies that a lump of matter has a higher energy content than the environment, whereas high entropy implies that the lump of matter and the environment are approaching equilibrium. Maximum entropy occurs when equilibrium has been reached. An analogy could be made with a well-organised library. In its normal working state, there would be a much greater concentration of books inside the library than outside; this state would be one of low entropy. If the books being removed were not returned, a state would be reached eventually when the concentration of books within the library would equal (for practical purposes) the concentration of books outside the library; this would be a state of maximum entropy. (One could question whether the library should be called a library in the latter state but this line of argument will not be pursued here. I will, however, return to it later.) It is relevant, when thinking of this analogy, to consider that the mechanism that allows the normal low entropy state to exist in the library is the activity of the librarians. In other words, energy is expended (by the librarians) to maintain the low entropy state and if the energy ceases to be expended, the library would eventually reach a state of maximum entropy with its books equally dispersed inside and outside it. This, I think, is a reasonable analogy to illustrate the concept of entropy without entering the realm of advanced mathematics that would not, in itself, clarify my argument.

We may now return to Schrödinger's original comments or observations, which, I think, are best summarised by saying that the feature common to all living entities is that they control their entropy with respect to their environment in such a way as to avoid the state of maximum entropy. This is not an abstract concept but a statement that can be verified by empirical observation of living entities ranging from the single-cell amoeba to multi-cellular organisms of great complexity, *e.g.* human beings. It is relatively straightforward to appreciate how a single-celled organism maintains a low entropy state; an intact cell membrane and the biochemical reactions associated with it allow a chemical concentration gradient to be maintained with respect to the outside environment. The answer in the case of human beings, however, is more complicated. In this case, not only must each cell maintain the low entropy state in a fashion similar to that of the single-celled organism, but in order for each individual specialised cell to achieve this state, the immediate outside environment must be maintained within a narrow range in terms of a number of physical and chemical variables, *e.g.* temperature, hydrogen ion and sodium ion concentration. This extra "layer" of maintenance is the penalty to be paid for the complexity of the whole entity and the specialisation of certain groups of cells within the entity. It is necessary, therefore, to maintain the physical and chemical properties of the fluids in which the cells lie within a narrow range in order to ensure the continued function of those cells. (The "narrowness" of the range to be maintained depends crucially upon the nature of the cells contained in that particular system.) This maintenance of the "internal milieu" of an entity is necessary in order that the cells maintain a low entropy state. In other words, in order for the cells of a multi-cellular organism, and in turn the organism as a whole, to maintain a low entropy state and, therefore, to survive it is necessary for the physical and chemical composition of the "internal milieu" of the organism to be maintained within narrow constraints. This maintenance of the "internal milieu" of the organism is referred to in humans (and other animals) as homeostasis. Therefore, in humans the ability to maintain a low entropy state and, therefore, to be classified as "living", using Schrödinger's criterion, is dependent on the continued ability to maintain homeostasis. This criterion, therefore, would seem to be the one that logically defines or separates the living from the non-living in human beings and forms the basis of the concept of death that I put forward and defend in this monograph.

Examination of the Features Possessed by an Animal such as a Human Being

For most people and for most of the time, there is no difficulty in answering the question "Is this individual alive?". Most people in these circumstances would seek the answers to the questions:
- Is the individual breathing spontaneously?
- Is the individual's heart still beating spontaneously?

The term "spontaneously" has been used here as a qualifier, since spontaneity of these two functions will be presumed or implicit in most ordinary concepts of life and death. Answers in the negative to both questions would lead to the statement that the individual was not alive; similarly, answers in the positive to both questions would produce a statement that the individual concerned was still alive. These steps have been used for some time by both lay and medically qualified persons to ascertain whether individuals were alive or dead (see chapter 1).

However, these tests are not infallible and Mant (1968) discusses this at some length. Even if the more sensational claims are excluded, there remain cases described by such eminent medical practitioners as Keith Simpson (1965, 1967). These cases, however, demonstrate not the fallibility of the criteria but the fallibility of the tests used to detect breathing and heartbeat. This fallibility was well known in earlier times and reference to it exists in Shakespeare (*Romeo and Juliet, Henry IV, King Lear*).

The question of the infallibility of the criteria is a separate one and is raised and severely tested by recent medical advances that enable machines (ventilators and cardiac by-pass pumps) to replace the functions of the lungs and the heart. Prior to the widespread use of ventilators, defibrillators, intensive-care units and cardiopulmonary resuscitation, failure of the cardiac, respiratory and neurological functions were closely linked. When one system failed, the other two inevitably failed as well. With the advent of these technologies, cardiac and respiratory function can be maintained for prolonged periods of time even in the presence of severe neurological deficit, *e.g.* unconsciousness. The end result is that the cardiac, respiratory and neurological functions are now no longer necessarily linked when one or other fails. It is entirely possible that an individual could be maintained on a ventilator or cardiac by-pass machines almost indefinitely and be able to conduct himself in an almost normal manner, especially if the present trend of miniaturisation of such machines continues. It is possible at the present time to implant a cardiac pacemaker to "drive" a damaged heart and to implant phrenic nerve stimulators to "drive" breathing. That people treated in such a manner are alive is, I think, beyond dispute, but what of the answers to the questions about their breathing and heartbeat? This demonstrates that the absence of spontaneous heartbeat and breathing are not sufficient conditions for death but they may, nonetheless, still be necessary conditions for death. What has been achieved is dissociation between the answers to the breathing/heartbeat status and the alive/dead status: it is possible to be alive and simultaneously have no spontaneous heartbeat or respiration. From this, I think that other criteria for life need to be promulgated. The morally important thing, which is contingent upon normal respiration and heartbeat, is the existence of a human being or person (however this may be conceived of philosophically). This latter is an area which I shall explore in greater depth in a later chapter, and about which I shall say nothing further at present.

In the rest of this chapter I would like to explore the possibility of establishing other criteria for life. Within the philosophical literature there is some discussion and disagreement about what constitutes a "person"

(Tooley, 1983; Harris, 1985a; Lizza, 1983; Carruthers, 1989; Englehardt, 1982; Crosby, 1993; Capron, 1987; Gervais, 1986a; Gervais, 1986b; Gillon, 1990; Dennett, 1981a, with a good summary by Evans (1996)) and, in order to proceed with my arguments, I will, for the present at least, use the term "human being". I should make it clear, at this point, that I view the question "Is this human being alive?" as simply one subset or species (as it were) of the more general question "Is this organism alive?". I view answers to the latter question (in terms of necessary and sufficient conditions for life) as applicable to the former question. I shall address, later in this chapter, the question of whether answers to the latter question, in terms of necessary and sufficient conditions for life can be considered as answers to the former question. In order to answer the question mentioned, that is "Is this organism alive?", there must be some criterion or criteria upon which the decision can be based. That is, there are some properties of living entities which are not shared with entities which are not living (Leibniz's rule: if A and B are not the same, then there must be at least one property they do not share). The phrase "not living" encompasses two classes of things, namely those "not living" things that were at some previous time "living" but which are "not living" now, and those "not living" things which were never "living". An example of the first group would be a dead animal or plant and the second group could be represented by a piece of stone (excluding sedimentary and carboniferous forms of stone).

What I am interested in is establishing the differences between the "living" group and the "not living"/"previously living" group, and there would be no point, therefore, in examining the "not living"/"never living" group. In other words, we should compare those things that are alive and those things that have been alive, and exclude examination of those things that have never been alive. The answer to the enquiry about the properties of "living" things is given by the study of physiology; Davson (1968) discusses this very topic and lists characteristics that "may, it is true, be mimicked by inanimate matter with or without man's ingenuity, but which, when taken together, leave the observer in little doubt that he is dealing with a living organism". These characteristics, according to Davson, are (summarised):

- Transformation of energy. This is, perhaps, the most distinctive feature of living organisms. Energy is needed for even the smallest of movements, for the maintenance of body temperature and for the production of electrical and osmotic potentials; even metabolism, the process by which energy is converted, requires energy to work.

- Organisation. As an organism becomes more complex, special structures are reserved for special functions and this exists both at the cellular level and at the level of the complete organism.
- Growth and reproduction. All living organisms grow and reproduce their own kind.
- Adaptation. All living organisms have the property of adaptation that can be defined as "the continuous adjustment of internal relations to external relations". A living organism is a highly unstable system that tends to undergo disintegration if its internal environment is changed beyond certain narrow limits.

If these four characteristics are examined closely, it can be seen that three of them, namely "transformation of energy", "organisation" and "adaptation" are such that they are all necessary for the maintenance of the internal environment of an organism, whereas the remaining characteristic "growth and reproduction" is concerned with the continuation of the species but is not necessary for the maintenance of the internal environment of the organism nor for the survival of any individual organism of any given species. These characteristics can, therefore, be summarised as two major characteristics of a living organism:

- capacity for the maintenance of the internal environment;
- capacity for growth and reproduction.

These exist to varying extents and are achieved by different methods in different organisms, but for the purposes of this discussion it is sufficient to establish that they do exist in all living organisms. It may be argued that only "warm-blooded" (homoiothermic) animals exhibit the capacity for homeostasis in that only they are able to maintain their body temperature constant within very narrow limits. However, to argue this would be mistaken since homeostasis is a matter of controlling a complex set of variables of which body temperature is only one, and not all solutions to the problem of homeostasis require precise regulation of body temperature within narrow limits or the use of the same mechanism to maintain control of any one variable. This use of different mechanisms to achieve the same end result is best illustrated by the different mechanisms of temperature control in different animals; when too warm, human beings (homoiothermic) sweat but dogs (also homoiothermic) pant since thick body hair precludes the mechanism of sweating whereas crocodiles (poikilothermic) move into the shade (a mechanism also available to human beings). All these mechanisms achieve the end result of maintaining body temperature within the appropriate normal range for the appropriate organism.

If we have the two characteristics for living animals just mentioned, we must ask whether both are essential in any one single animal prior to our being satisfied that the animal under discussion is alive. I would suggest that this is not the case. I would suggest that the second characteristic, namely the capacity for growth and reproduction, is essential for the survival of the species to which the animal under discussion belongs, but is not necessary for the continued survival of the individual animal. Therefore, it is entirely possible to have animals in existence, which do not have the capacity for reproduction, but which are unquestionably alive, for example the mule which is the off-spring of a male ass and a mare and which is sterile. Even if we are restricted to human beings, the creation and continued existence of clinics devoted entirely to infertility surely indicates that a significant proportion of the species is infertile; it would be difficult to maintain the stance that any infertile person is not alive. Therefore, while the capacity for reproduction is a characteristic that may be desirable in all living animals, it is not essential and certainly is not a criterion in the assessment of whether or not an animal is alive.

We must now examine, similarly, the other characteristic, namely the capacity for homeostasis. I have already argued that all living animals possess this, and I must now demonstrate that it is essential for the survival of the individual animal. Let us firstly examine again what we mean by the term "homeostasis". This is usually defined as the ability to maintain a constant internal environment despite variation in the external environment; it is usually possible only over a limited range of variation in the external environment, and if this range is exceeded the capacity for homeostasis is either reduced or lost. Essentially, therefore, the state produced by homeostasis is one in which there is a controlled difference between the organism and the environment in terms of certain parameters, for example temperature, concentration of various ions and organic/inorganic compounds.

If I am arguing that all living animals have the capacity for homeostasis, then it is germane to ask what happens when the limits of homeostasis are reached. What happens when an organism is, for example, warmed or cooled beyond the limits of homeostasis for that organism? Or what happens when the electrolyte imbalance in an organism is so great that it cannot be corrected by the organism? These are straightforward questions of fact and answers to them can be found in any standard textbook of physiology (if restriction is placed upon the nature of the organism). If the relatively narrow range of the limits of homeostasis is exceeded, the controlling mechanisms for each parameter that would normally be brought into play in an attempt to return the relevant parameter to the normal range, are no longer operative. When the disturbance to homeostasis is less, the controlling mechanism is operative and effective in most instances of disturbance. However, if the disturbance continues, the controlling mechanism becomes ineffective, although still operative. Once the disturbance exceeds the limits of homeostasis, the mechanism is no longer operative. For example, if hyperthermia (hyperpyrexia) is induced by excessive exposure to the sun, the normal mechanism for losing heat, namely sweating, no longer functions (that is, is no longer operative) and, if not treated externally, the temperature will continue to rise resulting in death. Similar results are obtained in hypothermia when shivering and pilo-erection (not very effective in the human) the normal homeostatic response to a fall in body temperature just do not occur when the limits of homeostasis are exceeded and the continuing reduction in body temperature eventually leads to death. Similar events unfold for the control of fluid balance, concentration of various ions and blood gas levels (pO_2 and pCO_2). (However, it is incidental to my main argument whether the various mechanisms continue to function and are overwhelmed or cease to function and are overwhelmed.)

In the preceding paragraph, I presented the scenario of what happens to an entity when the disturbance to homeostasis exceeds the limits of homeostasis for that entity. That is, the appropriate controlling mechanism becomes operative initially but later becomes inoperative. An implicit assumption in this scenario is that the controlling centre for homeostasis, wherever that may be anatomically in the entity, was initially intact prior to the disturbance. The question may reasonably be asked about the events that may happen when a disturbance to homeostasis occurs when the controlling centre for homeostasis is not functionally intact. In this case, any disturbance tending to push any parameter of homeostasis beyond the normal range for that parameter will not result in initiation of the normal mechanisms to restore it to the normal range; the end result will be that the parameter will very quickly exceed the normal range, and the result of this will be the same irrespective of the functional status of the controlling centre, *i.e.* death.

Therefore, intact homeostasis is required to maintain a variety of parameters within a relatively narrow range of values and since this maintenance within this relatively narrow range of values is necessary for living entities to continue living, it follows that control of homeostasis is necessary for living entities. That is, control of homeostasis is a necessary condition for life, as I have previously discussed the meaning of that phrase (see the first section of this chapter).

Examination of the Basic Common Features Existing in all Living Entities

What is being asked when a question is raised is about the necessary and sufficient conditions for life is an enquiry about the characteristic feature of life, that is about the feature or property of an entity that causes us to categorise that entity as being alive. What is it that causes us to say that a lump of matter is alive? Schrödinger (1944) put forward a tentative answer to this question that I have discussed in the first section of this chapter.

What I have argued in this section is that all living entities maintain a low entropy state; this low entropy state is a state never found in non-living entities. Therefore, it would seem to follow logically that a living human being or any other living entity is considered to be alive only for as long as the low entropy state is being maintained, *i.e.* for as long as homeostasis is being maintained in the case of human beings.

My line of argument in arriving at the necessary conditions for life may be criticised by some inasmuch as I have argued using an inductive argument to a necessary condition; this is generally held to be inappropriate or incorrect. My justification for such an approach is as follows. Let me consider an analogy using water. Initially we look at a variety of clear liquids and they appear identical. Closer examination reveals that not all the liquids are the same—some can be taken without ill effect (*e.g.* the one classified as water), but others cannot. Closer examination still allows us to discover the chemical composition of water (H_2O) and the chemical composition of, say, hydrochloric acid (HCl) another clear liquid. This allows a more precise classification—clear liquids with the chemical composition H_2O are classified as water. We have then reached a necessary condition for the classification of liquids into "water" or "not water". Similarly with entities—all may look alike initially but closer inspection reveals that some behave as described by Schrodinger (1944) inasmuch as they go on doing things much longer than we would expect or do things that we would not expect at all. These two groups of entities are then classified into "alive" and "not alive". Closer examination still (as with water) allows more detailed classification; those classified as alive do not appear to obey the 2nd Law of Thermodynamics and those classified as not alive do obey this Law. Those who do not obey this Law exhibit homeostasis and those who do not obey the Law do not exhibit homeostasis. As with water, we have reached a necessary condition; in the case of entities and the classification into "alive" or "not alive" the necessary condition is the presence or absence of homeostasis.

It may be argued that not all examples of life have been closely examined to reveal homeostasis and, therefore, strictly speaking the use of the term "necessary condition" is incorrect. Against this I would argue that no example of an entity that satisfies Schrödinger's description (1944) has ever been found that did not also exhibit homeostasis and, in addition, there are good theoretical reasons for thinking that an entity that satisfies Schrödinger's description and does not exhibit homeostasis will never be found. The reasoning is as follows:

- if an entity grows and moves, we classify it as alive;
- in order to grow and move the entity needs to acquire actively and store energy;
- only entities that do not obey the 2nd Law of Thermodynamics can actively acquire and store energy (by definition of the 2nd Law);
- if the 2nd Law of Thermodynamics is not obeyed, homeostasis is present.

Therefore, if an entity grows and moves (allowing us to classify it as alive without further examination) it will also have homeostasis. It is, therefore, reasonable to reach the necessary conditions for life by inductive reasoning on the grounds of lack of examples disproving the argument and good theoretical reasons for thinking that an example disproving the argument will never be found. Dennett is so convinced of this that he argues that one of the requirements for extraterrestrial life should such life exist, is that the organism will exhibit homeostasis (Dennett, 1995b).

Can There Be Sufficient Conditions for Life?

Both these arguments, that is the examination of the features possessed by an animal such as a human being and the examination of the basic common features existing in all living entities, lead me to the conclusion that control of an entity's internal environment is necessary for that entity to be classified as "alive". In other words, homeostasis is a necessary condition for life. However, the question about whether or not homeostasis is a sufficient condition for life has yet to be discussed. In order to answer this question, I would like to re-examine the idea put forward by Schrödinger (1944) that living entities maintain a state of low entropy and achieve this by expending energy. Let us consider such a single-cell entity and consider that it has lost the ability to reproduce (a single-cell entity such as an amoeba temporarily loses the ability to reproduce when there are insufficient nutrients). Since we have already said that the ability to reproduce, whilst necessary for the continuance of a species, is not necessary for the continued existence of any single member of that species, it follows that this single-cell entity should still be classified as alive despite the loss of reproduction.

To demonstrate that a condition is sufficient for life, it is necessary to demonstrate that an entity considered to be alive (this entity having control of homeostasis since it is a necessary condition for life) does nothing more than control its internal environment and thereby maintain its bodily integrity. In other words, for that entity specifying that it controls its internal environment and thereby maintains its bodily integrity is sufficient to say that the entity is alive. Now, if one considers a single-cell organism such as an amoeba, this organism normally has control of homeostasis and reproduces; however, reproduction occurs only under the correct circumstances and if these appropriate circumstances never occur in the life of such an organism then reproduction will not occur. Under these circumstances, the single-cell organism has all but one of the conditions put forward by Davson that "leave the observer in little doubt that he is dealing with a living organism" (Davson, 1968). It must be remembered at this point that the term "homeostasis" includes activities such as movement, engulfing and digesting food and avoiding other entities that may cause harm: these are all activities that are associated with living entities. An entity demonstrating such activities would be classified by *any* current criteria as being alive, despite the lack of the ability to reproduce. A single-cell organism such as an amoeba, without the ability to reproduce, exhibits all these features. In short, we would view the non-reproducing amoeba as alive because of the presence of the other features and despite the absence of the ability to reproduce. I have already argued that the other features are necessary for maintenance of homeostasis and, therefore, for the single-cell organism, specifying that control of homeostasis is present is sufficient to allow us to classify the organism as alive. In other words, for the single-cell organism, control of homeostasis is a sufficient condition for life.

From Single-cell Organisms to Human Beings

I have argued in the immediately preceding section that, for a single-cell organism, the control of homeostasis is a sufficient condition for life. The question to be addressed now is whether or not this argument can be extended to complex multi-cellular, multi-organ entities such as human beings. In other words, can this relationship between homeostasis and being classified as alive, which is reasonable for a single-cell organism, be taken as a general relationship for all living entities irrespective of complexity? There are two positions that could be adopted:

- Accept that, by extension, life is present in more complex organisms when the criteria for life used in the single-cell organism are present in the more complex organism, that is the control of homeostasis. Acceptance of this would mean that control of homeostasis, in addition to being a necessary and sufficient condition for life in single-cell organisms would also be a necessary and sufficient condition for life in more complex organisms including human beings.
- Argue that in more complex organisms, including human beings, life is present when and only when other criteria or conditions are met in addition to the condition of the control of homeostasis. This position means that whilst control of homeostasis is both a necessary and sufficient condition for life in a single-cell organism, it is only a necessary condition but not a sufficient condition for life in more complex organisms including human beings.

The first of these two proposals has two positive features. Firstly, under this proposal, the concept of life is a straightforward one and secondly the concept of life is uniform throughout the whole range of entities that we would consider to be alive. In other words, the concept of life is uniform in all living entities. If death is viewed as the absence of life, it follows from this uniform concept of life that there would also be a uniform concept of death. In other words, the terms "life" and "death" would retain their respective uniform meanings irrespective of the organism to which they were applied. The simplicity of the concept of life under this proposal and the uniformity or constancy of meaning throughout the whole range of entities considered to be alive are features of the first proposal that I view as very positive.

In the case of the second proposal, that is that life is present in more complex organisms when and only when other criteria or conditions, in addition to the condition of control of homeostasis, are present, the concept of death is not straightforward and creates a problem with the meaning of the term "life" and, consequently, with the term "death". Under this proposal, life would be present in single-cell organism when homeostasis was present, when homeostasis and criterion X is present in a more complex organism and when homeostasis and criterion Y (Y may or may not contain X as a subset) is present in another, different more complex organism. In other words, the term "life" would have different meanings depending upon the complexity of the organism to which it was being applied. Since the variations in complexity between different organisms are extremely large, the end result of this approach would be to produce an extremely large number of meanings for the term "life". Of course, it follows that there would be an equally large number of meanings for the term "death". I can see no rational basis for this approach; the terms "life" and "death" should have the same meaning regardless of the organism to which they are applied. Dennett expresses a similar opinion when he says "human beings, as mammals, must fall under the principles of biology that cover all mammals. Mammals, in turn, are composed of molecules, which must obey the laws of chemistry, which in turn must answer to the regularities of the underlying physics" (Dennett, 1995c). Dennett is suggesting that we view human beings with the same criteria as we view other mammals on the basis that all organisms must obey the rules of chemistry and physics—there are no exceptions for human beings. Lamb (1985) expresses the same opinion when he says

> "Death, so defined as the irreversible loss of the function of the organism as a whole, is a singular concept. It does not make sense to speak of one kind of death for humans and another kind for other life forms."

This is a line of argument that I shall return to later.

As Dennett (1995c) points out, all mammals including human beings and implicitly all other animals are subject to the same rules of chemistry and physics without exception. It is implicit in the application of the same rules of physics and chemistry to all animals (and to physical and chemical processes *in vitro*) that a given term will have the same meaning in relation to the relevant physical or chemical process within an animal (and to the same physical and chemical process *in vitro*). In other words, terms such as acidification or phosphorylation have the same meaning irrespective of the animal in which the process has occurred (and irrespective of whether the process is *in vivo* or *in vitro*). I would argue that we should be able to assume that the meanings for the processes that are common to living organisms are constant, irrespective of the complexity of the animal. In other words, if we were to say that a human being metabolised a certain food and then used the term "metabolise" in relation to another animal or organism, we should use the same meaning for the term and not have to re-define "metabolise" for each and every organism to which we apply it. By the same argument, if the term "homeostasis" means "control of the internal environment" in a single-cell organism, then it has the same meaning for all living organisms, including human beings. If I argue that death is the permanent loss of the ability to control the internal environment when applied to a single-cell organism then the term "death", when used in reference to more complex organisms including human beings, should still be the permanent loss of the ability to control the internal environment.

Against my argument there could be raised the counter-argument that while this relationship between maintenance of the internal environment and being classified as alive is acceptable for single-cell organisms and other organisms of limited complexity, the argument is not acceptable for human beings; human beings are more complex and are of more value (to other human beings, although not necessarily because of their complexity) than other organisms. This argument would mean that while control of homeostasis is both necessary and sufficient for the categorisation of single-cell organisms and some other (as yet unspecified) more complex organisms as alive, the control of homeostasis would be necessary but not sufficient for the categorisation of yet other, still more complex organisms as alive. The usual reason put forward for this suggested difference is that we value the more complex organisms more than we value single-cell organisms; this is the basic approach taken by those who advocate a "higher function" approach to the concept of death (Gervais, 1986; Veatch, 1975; Beecher, 1968; Green and Wickler, 1980). This group advocates a concept of death that can be applied only to human beings (see chapter 2 for discussion). My rebuttal of this counter-argument that a special case should be made for human beings simply because they are human beings is three-fold:

- The selection for special treatment of human beings simply on the basis of membership of the group of organisms referred to as human beings is not a morally sound selection. There is not much more that can be said about such a selection on such a basis.
- Leaving aside the question of the moral basis of the selection of human beings for special treatment as outlined above, the selection process itself does not include all human beings and, indeed, excludes a significant number of human beings. The number and nature of the human beings excluded by such a process is totally dependent upon the precise criteria used in the selection process; different criteria are used by different members of the group (Gervais, 1986; Veatch, 1975; Beecher, 1968; Green and Wickler, 1980). However, the various criteria exclude anencephalic new-borns, new-borns generally, the

comatose, those in the persistent vegetative state, foetuses and the severely mentally disabled.
- Careful enquiry must be made about the precise basis for the value put upon human beings by other human beings, assuming that the first paragraph above does not apply. A variety of authors have put forward a range of criteria upon which the value of a human being can be based (Gervais, 1986; Veatch, 1975; Beecher, 1968; Green and Wickler, 1980). However, it should be remembered that these authors are discussing value and the features of human beings (or, more precisely, of some human beings as I have indicated in the second paragraph above) that we should value; they are not discussing the presence or absence of organic life. Lamb (1985) summarises this well by saying:

> "It may be that humans are the only species with a sense of personal identity, but the loss of this sense should not imply a different form of death for humans. A human being without identity is just as alive as any other living being."

Their arguments and discussion are, therefore, not entirely relevant to the question of whether or not organic life in a human being should be viewed as the same as organic life in any other living organism including single-cell organisms.

The criticism of my argument that all living organisms should be viewed with the same definition or meaning of life and death is based, therefore, on the argument that human beings are of more value than other living entities. However, it seems that the features of human beings (or some human beings, as I have already pointed out) that give them this value are features that are present (in some human beings) in addition to the presence of organic life. Essentially, my counter-argument against this criticism is that the definition or meaning of a term applied to a process (namely, life or death) common to all living organisms should not be changed for one species of living organism because of the presence of other features unique to that species (but not present in all members of that species). Whilst conceding that human beings *may* be of more value than other living organisms, I would contend that the definition or meaning of the terms applied to common processes remain uniform irrespective of the species to which they are applied. In other words, the terms "life" and "death" should mean the same for all living organisms.

I have now argued that if we accept that life is present in single-cell organisms when homeostasis is present then we should accept that life is present in more complex organisms, including human beings, when homeostasis is present. I have also argued that, if the presence of homeostasis is a sufficient condition for life in a single-cell organism, then it should be accepted as a sufficient condition for life in more complex organisms, including human beings.

Summary

I have argued in this chapter that there can be necessary and sufficient conditions for life. I have also presented arguments that the control of the internal environment of an entity is both a necessary and sufficient condition for the classification of that entity as "alive", irrespective of the complexity of the entity. The necessary and sufficient conditions for life are that maintenance of the internal environment occurs.

References

Beecher, H.K. (1968), "A definition of irreversible coma", *J. American Med. Ass.*, vol. 205, pp. 337-340.
Capron, A. (1987), "Anencephalic donors: separate the dead from the dying", *Hastings Center Report*, vol. 17(1), pp. 5-9.
Carruthers, P. (1989), *Introducing persons*, Routledge, London, p. 234.
CRC (1979), *Handbook of Chemistry and Physics*, R.C. Weast, and M.J. Astle (eds.), Chemical Rubber Co. Publ., 1979, pp. F104-5.
Crosby, J.F. (1993), "The personhood of the human embryo", *J. Medicine and Philosophy*, vol. 18(4), pp. 399-417.
Davson, H. (1968) in H. Davson, M.G. Eggleton, *Principles of Human Physiology*, 14th ed., Churchill Livingstone, London.
Dennett, D.C. (1995a), *Darwin's dangerous idea*, Penguin Books, London, p. 127.
Dennett, D.C. (1995b), *Darwin's dangerous idea*, Penguin Books, London, p. 81.
Dennett, D. (1981), *Brainstorms: philosophical essays on mind and psychology*, Harvester Press, Brighton, pp. 269-271.
Englehardt, H.T. (1982), "Concepts of personhood", in T.L. Beauchamp and L. Walters (eds), *Contemporary Issues in Bioethics*, 1st ed., Wadsworth, Belmont, pp. 97-98.
Evans, M. (1996), "Some ideas of the person", in D. Greaves and H. Upton (eds.), *Philosophical problems in health care*, Avebury, Aldershot, pp. 23-35.
Gervais, K.G. (1986a), *Redefining death*, Yale Univ. Press, New Haven, p. 157.
Gervais, K.G. (1986b), *Redefining death*, Yale Univ. Press, New Haven, p. 181.
Gervais, K.G. (1986c), *Redefining death*, Yale Univ. Press, New Haven, pp. 223-229.
Gillon, R. (1990), "Death", *J. Medical Ethics*, vol. 16(1), pp. 3-4.
Green, M.B. and Wikler, D. (1980), "Brain death and personal identity", *Philosophy and Public Affairs*, vol. 9, pp. 105-133.
Harris, J. (1985), *The value of life*, Routledge, London, pp. 9-10.
Lamb, D. (1985), *Death, brain death and ethics*, State Univ. of New York Press, Albany, p. 93.

Lizza, J. (1993), "Persons and death", *J. Medicine and Philosophy*, vol. 18(4), pp. 351-374.

Mant, A.K. (1968), "The medical definition of death", in A.K. Mant, *Man's concern with death*, Hodder & Stoughton, London, pp. 13-24.

Schrödinger, E. (1944), *What is life?*, Cambridge Univ. Press, Cambridge, (reprinted 1992, version referred to), pp. 69-75.

Shakespeare W. *Henry IV*, Part II.

Shakespeare W. *King Lear*, act 5, sc. 3.

Shakespeare W. *Romeo and Juliet*, act 5, sc. 3.

Simpson, K. (1965), *Taylor's Principles and Practice of Medical Jurisprudence*, 12th ed., Churchill Livingstone, London.

Simpson, K. (1967), *Abbotempo*, vol. 3, p. 22.

Tooley, M. (1983), *Abortion and infanticide*. Clarendon Press, Oxford, p. 51.

Veatch, R.M. (1975), "The whole brain oriented concept of death: an outmoded philosophical formulation", *J. Thanatology*, vol. 3, pp. 13-30.

7 Justification for the Adoption of a Biological Concept of Death

*"Leaving one still with the intolerable wrestle
With words and meanings"*
T.S. Elliot *Four Quartets* "East Coker" pt. 2

Introduction

In chapter 6 I argued that there could be necessary and sufficient conditions for life and suggested that only the maintenance of the internal environment satisfied both these conditions. This maintenance of the internal environment can also be referred to as the maintenance of bodily integrity or the maintenance of homeostasis (this latter term being in common use with reference to human beings). In this chapter I will put forward arguments to defend my concept of death as the permanent loss of the ability to maintain bodily integrity or, in the human being, the permanent loss of the control of homeostasis.

From the age of Francis Bacon, there has been a general feeling that there was no limit to science—that there was no question that would not inevitably succumb to scientific enquiry. Peter Medawar (1984) gives a short but lucid account of this phase in the history of science. However, he argues that there are questions "that science cannot answer and that no conceivable advance of science could empower it to answer". Popper (discussed by Medawar) also argues that there are "ultimate questions" that science will never be able to answer, *e.g.* "What are we all here for?" and "What is the point of living?"

If we accept that there exists a type of question that science cannot answer, then we must enquire about the difference between this type of question and the type of question that science has been asking and answering with spectacular success since the time of Bacon. Questions in science are asked and the answers are suggested in the form of hypotheses that, importantly, can be tested by empirical observation. While methodologists may differ in their interpretation of the process of evaluating hypotheses, there is no doubt that, in science, all hypotheses must be evaluated. As Medawar points out (1984) most of "the day-to-day business of science consists in making observations and doing experiments bearing upon the acceptance or modification of hypotheses". If we ask an analogous question of the answers offered to the "ultimate questions" of Popper, we find that none can be verified by empirical observation as employed in science. With regard to hypotheses in general, Kant expressed his demand for verification as "it must be unconditionally true of any hypotheses that it could possibly be true" (discussed by Medawar), *i.e.* any hypomonograph must be verifiable in principle. This, of course, is not possible with any reasonable answers to the "ultimate questions". It follows that the answers to these questions cannot lie within the realm of scientific enquiry.

Medawar raises the possibility that the answer to questions such as "How did everything begin?" may be empirical in nature and, therefore, be amenable to scientific enquiry and proof. He refutes this suggestion on the basis that we cannot have empirical awareness of a frontier between being and nothingness without having an empirical awareness of what lies on the other side of it. Whereas this side of this particular frontier poses no special problem, for we can be aware of that which is being, there can be no empirical awareness of nothingness. The result is, Medawar suggests, that if such a frontier exists, it cannot exist in the domain of scientific enquiry. If science cannot answer questions such as these, then to whom do we turn in order to receive an answer? Traditionally, answers to questions such as these have been sought in the realms of religion or philosophy. However, within the major Western religions there is a tendency to offer answers that are either "revealed" truths or reiterations of the statements of earlier religious thinkers; these answers are then treated as though they were fact rather than opinion (however well considered the opinion may be). Such answers can be a little incongruent with the everyday world of experience and common sense and are consequently rejected by many. An example would be the insistence by the major Western religions that death of an individual occurs when the soul leaves the body. Medicine has attempted to accommodate this concept as I have discussed in the chapter on the reasons for rejecting the current concepts of death (chapter 4) but has achieved only a mismatched amalgam of criteria for death that are not logically derived from the concept of death. Attempts within the discipline of philosophy to answer such questions have, largely, a correspondence with real life and, as a direct result, have found adherents among those who cannot accept theological explanations to this group of questions. While the opinions of Jonas (1974), Beecher (1968), Gervais (1986a) and Veatch (1975, 1989) on the concept of death are disparate in the extreme, they all have the advantage over the Western theological concept of death that the concept of death each holds is logically considered and not "revealed wisdom" and can produce logically derived criteria for death that are of use in the appropriate practical setting.

Theoretical Arguments

Having argued that there is a group of questions that cannot reasonably be asked of science and should more properly be addressed to philosophy, I must now ask if the question with which I am grappling is a member of this group. The question under discussion is "What is death?". This would certainly seem to fit the description given by Medawar (discussed earlier) concerning a frontier beyond which there is nothingness. (Various religions might wish to argue that beyond death is not nothingness, but the state they believe to exist beyond death is a "revealed truth" and not amenable to the rigour of scientific proof, as I have argued earlier. There are no empirical observations that indicate the existence of anything, in terms of conscious experience, beyond death.) Nagel also takes the view that "death is nothing, and final" (Nagel, 1986). Hence there is a *prima facie* case that the answer to my question lies within the realm of philosophy and not science. Becker (1988a) summarises this well when he says that there are two propositions about the boundaries of life, *viz.*
- there is no decisive way to define, in purely biological terms, either the point at which a human life begins, or the point at which it ends;
- in any case, if the end points are going to be used as moral divides, they should be defined in terms of morally relevant characteristics, not purely biological ones.

However, like Becker, I wish to argue against these propositions and for the position that the answer to the question "What is death?" can be answered, at least in part, in biological terms. That is to say, I am suggesting that an end point that marks a moral divide can be defined, at least in part, in biological terms. Death is the frontier between two states, namely the "being" and the "has-been". Becker (1988b) summarises his argument as follows:
- exit from the class of human beings is a process;
- the exit process is at least in part a biological one;

- the completion of the biological part of the exit process is a necessary condition for the completion of the exit process per se.

Despite the frequent use of the phrase "at least in part", Becker proceeds to argue that the death of a human being, *i.e.* the divide between "being" and "has-been", should be viewed entirely as a biological event. It would seem that he has moved imperceptibly from a "weak" stance to a "strong" stance with regard to the biological concept of death. (It is also worth noting that Becker argues that "brain death" is neither a definition of, nor a criterion for, the "being"/"has-been" frontier.) I would like to argue for the "strong" position in relation to the biological concept of death, that is that the concept of death could be expressed totally in biological terms despite the role played by death in a moral divide. However, I would like to begin by examining the "weak" position, *i.e.* that the concept of death can be expressed, only in part, in biological terms. The logical result of the stance that only part of the concept of death can be expressed in biological terms is that the other part must be expressed in non-biological terms. If this is the case, then what are these non-biological terms to be? This point is raised by Gervais (1986b) as part of her criticism of Becker's argument, and is correctly interpreted as a point of weakness in that argument. If the biological part of the concept of death is a necessary condition, then what constitutes the remaining part must be "non-biological". If the "non-biological" terms are to be included in the concept of death, are we not in danger of attempting to conjoin two different languages in an attempt to describe the same event? The concept of death can be expressed in the different terms of different languages, for instance:

- religious: the loss of the soul from the body (Pope Pius, 1957);
- philosophical: the loss of consciousness and those features peculiar to human life (Gervais, 1986b, as an example of a group who hold similar views);
- biological: the loss of the ability to maintain bodily integrity (my own).

(These examples are not intended to be exhaustive, merely illustrative.) While it is permissible to express the concept of death (or any other concept) in any one of these separate terms or languages, it is not permissible to employ more than one language at any one time (Weissmann, 1946). This latter manoeuvre is exactly what Becker suggests we do, namely, frame part of the concept of death in the terms of one language (biological) and another part of the concept in the terms of another, different, language (non-biological). It is probably best to illustrate what Becker is trying to do by means of an analogy. If we consider the appearance of mankind on earth, we find that this can be described in two significantly different ways, namely in terms of religion (whether Christianity or Islam is immaterial for my purpose) and in terms of science according to the theory of evolution. In the language of the religious explanation, mankind was created as an act of a supreme being and in the language of science mankind slowly evolved from other animals; the language of one does not admit of the ideas or language of the other. To attempt to explain the appearance of mankind on earth in terms of the languages of both religion and science simultaneously would not be feasible since the languages have nothing in common. This, essentially, is what Becker is suggesting should be done with the concept of death. Perhaps an even better analogy would be with the study of the stars and their movements. These matters can be described either in the language of astronomy that is a science-based discipline or in the language of astrology that is, perhaps, less scientifically based. I think that anyone who tried to discuss the stars and planets in a way that combined these two, quite separate, languages would not be taken seriously by members of either camp; one of the appropriate languages should be used but not both simultaneously. Again, Becker would have us adopt a concept of the heavens that would be described in an amalgam of both languages. With regard to the study of the heavens as with the concept of death, one language should be adopted and the concept framed only in that language. (A quite separate issue, I think, is whether or not one language can be translated into another as can be done with everyday languages in use in different parts of the world, for example English translated into French or German translated into Mandarin Chinese. However, despite this translation facility between the languages being possible, ideas are expressed totally in one language (we can ignore the small phrases borrowed from one language and inserted into another, for example *"raison d'être"*, since they express an idea not easily expressed in the language into which they have been transplanted and, in addition, constitute only a minute fraction of any language into which they are inserted). In addition, it is commonly accepted that something of the idea expressed in the original language can be lost or distorted in such translations. Similarly with the concept of death: it is perfectly valid to have three (or more) concepts of death in different languages, but it is not possible to merge two (or more) of these concepts as Becker is attempting to do when he adopts the "weak" stance with regard to the biological concept of death. Weissmann discusses this inability to express an idea or concept in more than one language simultaneously, and concludes that a concept can only be expressed in one language and not in a mixture of two or more languages (Weissmann, 1946). Hence Becker is doomed to failure by adopting this approach of trying to express a concept of death simultaneously in more that one language.

I am, therefore, forced to reject the "weak" and examine the "strong" position. This states that the concept of death can be expressed entirely in biological terms. (This should not be taken to mean that the other concepts of death summarised earlier are of no value. I shall return to this later.) My reasons for adopting a purely biological concept of death can be summarised as follows:
- all human beings are members of that class of beings called animals;
- all animals die;
- since death is common to all animals, the concept of death should be the same for all animals;
- an identical concept of death for all animals cannot be achieved in a language other than the biological one.

I will now expand on these points.

That human beings are members of the class of being commonly referred to as animals would seem to be a matter of common observation and beyond dispute. Empirical observation suggests that human beings have many features, both anatomical and physiological, in common with animals. While it seems to be generally accepted that human beings are descended from the apes, this is a scientific theory and indisputable proof of the theory is lacking. A recent publication argued that this theory is grossly defective (Milton), and that the theory of evolution (as put forward by Darwin in the Origin of Species) is not scientifically founded. Despite this, however, mainstream scientific thought holds that the basic tenets of Darwin's theory are correct and that, from the scientific viewpoint, human being are no different from other animals, a stance cogently argued for by Rachels (1991). I shall, therefore, accept that human beings are animals.

The second point, that is that all animals die, is a statement that can be made *a priori*. While this is true for any multi-cell animal from empirical observation, the suggestion could be made that the statement that all animals die does not apply to single-cell organisms such as amoeba. The basis for this assertion is that these single-cell organisms reproduce asexually by simple division after duplication of their genetic material; the resultant two organisms are genetically identical. Therefore, destruction of one leaves intact an exact copy of the original. In some sense we might think it could be said of the original that it has not died. This is a fallacy created by the confusion between what constitutes an entity and the genetic material contained within an entity. While it is true, in the circumstances described above, that the original genetic material still exists in the survivor of the two off-spring, it is an error to refer to this as the genetic material remaining "alive". The genetic material is still in existence, that is all. The term "alive" should be more properly applied to living entities, and not to inanimate organic material. If we call the original single-cell organism "O" and the two off-spring "A" and "B", and I choose to destroy "A" after "O" has divided into "A" and "B", then "B" remains alive with the original genetic material from "O" intact. However, "A" is dead. If, however, after "O" has divided into "A" and "B" both "A" and "B" are allowed to live, they will become different organisms as a result, for example, of different environments. Therefore, separate and different single-cell organisms exist neither of which resembles the original ("O"), although the genetic material in each is the same. Therefore, even in the case of single-cell organisms, death of the organism occurs.

My third point is that since all animals die, there is a strong *prima facie* case for the concept of death to be the same in all cases (see chapter 6). I have argued in the preceding paragraph that all animals die, that is they cross the boundary between "being" and "has been" in Becker's terms (1988a). Since all animals must, at some time, reach this boundary, and we define this boundary for all animals outside the species Homo sapiens in biological terms, it would seem logical to define that same boundary for members of the species Homo sapiens in the same terms, *i.e.* in biological terms. This, in fact, is the state of affairs that has existed from historical times, namely that human beings *and other animals* were considered to be dead if there was no heartbeat and no spontaneous breathing. In other words, a common set of criteria for death was used. I would like to suggest that this uniformity of concept be retained, especially in the absence of any convincing argument to the contrary. Many such as Veatch (1975), Beecher (1969) and Gervais (1986a) would argue that human beings are not mere animals and that as a group have features that distinguish us, in a morally important way from other animals. They would argue that the concept of death for the species Homo sapiens should be based on these morally important differences; I have considered these points at some depth in the chapter on the reasons for rejection of present concepts of death (chapter 4).

Concerning my fourth point, if a uniform concept of death is to be adopted, then we must ask in what language this concept can be expressed. I have suggested earlier that the concept of death could be expressed in at least three different languages, *i.e.* religious, philosophical and biological, and I shall now argue that it is possible to have a uniform concept of death, applicable to humans and other animals alike, only if that concept is expressed in the language of biology. If we examine the religious concept of death as expounded by Pope Pius XII (1957), we find that death of a human being occurs when the soul leaves the body. I would have to agree with Pallis (1983) that such a concept would make it "difficult to identify this particular state or to formulate relevant criteria", but that is not the question raised here. The present question is whether this concept of death is unique to human beings or could be a uniform concept covering all animals. The answer to the question hinges on the fact (or, more correctly, belief?) that the soul must leave the body for death to occur. It follows that if the animal in question (*i.e.* non-human) did not possess a soul, then, in terms of this concept, death could not occur. Since, as I have already argued, death occurs for all animals without exception, then either all animals possess souls or this concept (that is, the religious one) cannot be extended to animals other than human beings. Thomas Aquinas (discussed in Russell (1984)), a philosopher of great renown in the Roman Catholic faith, held that animals have souls but that, unlike the souls of men, they were not immortal. It would seem, therefore, that it is at least possible that the religious concept of death could be applied to all animals. There is a problem here, however; if the animal (that is, non-human) soul is not immortal then the implication is that the soul dies with the body. There are several possible explanations for this. Firstly, the soul does not leave the body, and therefore dies when the body dies. This poses a major problem because if the soul does not leave the body, then according to the concept of death, death has not occurred: immortality is the logical result of this explanation and since empirical observation dictates that this is not the case then this explanation must be rejected. Secondly, it is possible to argue that the soul does, in fact, leave the body thereby causing the death of the animal, and immediately thereafter dies itself. This explanation satisfies the condition that the soul is not immortal and also that the soul leaving the body has caused death. I would suggest that this concept of death is not capable of being a uniform one and that a uniform concept of death cannot be expressed in the language of the western religions since they share this concept of death.

What is possible with the language of philosophy? Although there are differences between the concepts of death advocated by Gervais (1986b), Beecher (1969), Pallis (1983) and Veatch (1975), all suggest that the permanent loss of the capacity for consciousness should be viewed as death. What they have in common is that they all argue that the possession of the capacity for consciousness (or the capacity for some other function that depends on the capacity for consciousness) is an essential, ontological difference between human beings and other animals. If this latter statement is to be accepted, then it follows that other non-human animals, which do not possess the capacity for consciousness, cannot be encompassed by any concept of death that includes the permanent loss of that capacity. While other philosophers such as Singer argue that some animals exhibit consciousness (Singer, 1988) and could thereby be encompassed by the concept of death promulgated by Gervais (1986), Beecher (1969), Pallis (1983) and Veatch (1975), this is not accepted by these philosophers who obviously take the view that animals do not exhibit consciousness and cannot, therefore, be encompassed by their concepts of death. Hence, this philosophical stance produces a concept of death that can, by definition, be applied only to human beings and cannot become a uniform concept of death.

Lastly, we come to the concept of death expressed in biological terms. The biological concept of death for which I would like to argue is that the permanent loss of the ability to maintain bodily integrity entails death, but I will mention other biological concepts of death later; it is only relevant, here, to argue for a concept which is essentially biological and to discuss the variety of such concepts later. I have already argued:

- (in chapter 6) that empirical observation indicates that all animals maintain, by a variety of means, their bodily integrity;
- (in this chapter) that all animals die, again from empirical observation that all biological systems cease to exist.

I would further argue that, since human beings and other animals are biological systems and will therefore cease to exist (*i.e.* die), then it is at least logical that this death should be expressed in biological terms. Since death is common to human beings and animals, it would follow that a function, the loss of which would uniquely constitute death, must be common to human beings and animals. While we cannot be certain about whether animals, in general, possess selected functions such as consciousness or self-consciousness, nor be certain as to the behaviour of an animal soul, we would like to be certain about death; it follows that this function (the permanent loss of which would constitute death) is something about which we should be certain. I have argued that this function must be one of which we can be certain and, simultaneously, be one possessed by human beings and animals. This means that, by exclusion, this property must be a biological one. There is nothing new in this advocacy of the use of a biological definition of death, indeed, a biological definition of death

has been in use for a long time; death of a human or of an animal has been pronounced when there has been
- prolonged absence of breathing;

and
- cessation of heartbeat.

Therefore, there is nothing innovative about the use of a biological definition of death that is applicable to both humans and non-humans.

While these arguments for the selection of a biological concept of death support my contention that the biological concept is the concept that should be adopted, there are other reasons for the adoption of the biological concept of death. Both Pallis (1983) and Lamb (1985) have argued that criteria for death only

> "have meaning if they can be shown to be logically derived from the appropriate concept of death. It is therefore meaningless to use 'free-floating criteria' that are not derived from a clearly determined concept of death".

It should be borne in mind that derivation of a set of criteria for death from a concept of death does not automatically ensure the adequacy, philosophically, of the concept. For example, Pallis (1983) quotes a concept of death in use in the Middle Ages, namely the entering of certain monastic orders, from which criteria could logically be derived: a concept such as this, even with any related criteria, can be viewed as referring to death only in a metaphorical sense. I am concerned with death in the literal sense and concepts of death like the one just discussed are of peripheral interest only.

Practical Arguments

I would like to extend the argument of Pallis (1983) and Lamb (1985), relating to the criteria for death, to the concept of death. That is, I would like to put forward the argument that just as "free-floating criteria" are meaningless, then "free-floating concepts" are equally meaningless. By the phrase "free-floating concepts", I mean concepts from which it is not possible to produce criteria (and it follows that if criteria cannot be produced, then tests cannot be derived since there would be no criteria on which to base them). Any concept of death from which criteria could not logically be derived would be in a vacuum, unconnected to any logical derivation. If "criteria without concept" is meaningless according to Pallis and Lamb, then I would suggest that "concept without criteria" is unusable in the present context of practical application of a concept of death. With this in mind, let us examine the three main concepts of death discussed earlier, *i.e.* religious, philosophical and biological. The religious concept of death as put forward by Pope Pius XII (1957) is that death occurs when the soul departs from the body. While Aquinas (discussed in Russell (1984)) describes in some detail exactly what constitutes a soul, it must be remembered that the soul is not a physical entity (by definition) and that the process of the soul leaving the body is not a process that lends itself to empirical observation: no-one has observed or seen a soul. This leads to great problems in the development of criteria based on this concept of death, a point expressed by Pallis in his monograph (1983). Pope Pius XII seems content to leave the determination of death to medically qualified personnel (Pope Pius, 1957) using whatever criteria they think fit; he has not indicated any criteria derived from the concept he has just advocated. Therefore, any criteria used by the medical profession will not be linked logically to the religious concept of death; they will either be "free-floating" or linked logically to another, non-religious concept of death. In either event, the concept expounded has not resulted in a logically derived set of criteria for death.

Can the philosophical concept of death produce logically derived criteria? The concepts put forward by Gervais (1986a), Veatch (1975), Beecher (1969) and Pallis (1983) can certainly lead to logically derived criteria as all four philosophers have demonstrated. All four suggest that consciousness, or a feature for which consciousness is a necessary condition such as self-consciousness, is of prime concern and all include the permanent loss of consciousness in their respective concepts of death. However, there is a problem with the use of consciousness as a criterion for death. The problem is that there is no agreed definition of consciousness. Different authors attach different meanings to the term and there are some who would argue that animals possess consciousness (Singer, 1988), whilst others would hold equally strong views that animals do not possess consciousness (Gervais, 1986b; Veatch, 1975; Beecher, 1969). What we have, therefore, is:

- a multiplicity of meanings for this term "consciousness";
- uncertainty about which animals possess or demonstrate consciousness; this uncertainty derives partly from (1) above and partly from the general inability to assess consciousness in some animals, *e.g.* earthworms.

Using the presence or absence of consciousness in the criteria for death would be akin to saying that A is dead if a state X exists in relation to A, but without providing an agreed definition of the state X. In other words, A could be simultaneously alive and dead by the same criterion simply because of a multiplicity of meanings of the terms in the criterion. This, assuredly, is not a desirable state of affairs!

Another problem with the use of consciousness as a criterion for death, apart from the multiplicity of meanings, is that there are degrees of consciousness or, to use more accurate terminology, degrees of consciousness are recognised by practising neurologists and neurosurgeons (Teasdale, 1974). Even outside that esoteric world, it is generally recognised that degrees of consciousness exist, for example sleeping is not the same as permanent coma and there is "deep" and "light" sleep. If the loss of consciousness is to be used as a criterion for death, then which level of consciousness is to be used? The answer given by proponents of consciousness as a criterion is that the loss of consciousness must be permanent. Certainly one could not rationally object to the insertion of this qualifying term. However, herein lies another problem with the use of permanent unconsciousness as the sole criterion of death, that is the practical difficulty of establishing that unconsciousness is permanent. The proponents of the use of consciousness as the sole criterion of death have taken as the paradigm state the clinical condition commonly known as the persistent vegetative state; they argue that this state of permanent unconsciousness should be viewed as death. There are two points to be noted here. Firstly, the there is an elision from the term "persistent" to the term "permanent"; these two terms are not synonymous for there is nothing in the term "persistent" to indicate irreversibility, whereas the term "permanent" could be replaced in all of its uses by the term "irreversible". Therefore there has been a subtle re-definition of the clinical condition of persistent vegetative state without presentation of data to support such a re-definition. Indeed such data as exist indicate that in a significant number of cases of persistent vegetative state recovery to a conscious state can occur (Andrews, 1992; Steinbock, 1989). Secondly, there is the practical difficulty, mentioned earlier, of establishing the permanence of any period of unconsciousness; this is well illustrated by the data from Andrews (Andrews, 1992). These findings illustrate the great difficulty encountered in establishing whether or not a particular state of unconsciousness is permanent. Therefore, while the state of permanent unconsciousness might be an acceptable criterion of death to some at a theoretical level, the use of unconsciousness as the sole criterion of death at a practical level is unsound.

With regard to a biological concept of death, we must ask the same question that we have asked of the other concepts of death, that is whether or not it is possible to logically derive a set of criteria from such a concept. Certainly if one examines the particular biological concept of death that I advocate, *i.e.* that the permanent loss of the ability to maintain bodily integrity constitutes death, then it is possible to derive a set of criteria for death. If it is accepted that the permanent loss of the ability to maintain bodily integrity is a valid concept of death, then the criterion derived from that concept would be the permanent loss of the control of homeostasis (if we restrict the present discussion to human beings). Since homeostasis consists of the control of functions such as temperature, fluid balance, blood pressure and acid-base balance (Davson, 1968; Lewis, 1968; Macknight, 1994) then the tests for death derived from this criterion would be tests for the control of these functions (I discuss this again in chapter 11).

Summary

I have argued in this chapter that it is valid to use a biological concept of death. I have also argued that the religious and philosophical concepts of death are flawed in that neither seems to produce workable criteria for death. On this basis I have argued that the only reasonable concepts of death to use are biological. I have also put forward the criterion and tests for death logically derived from my own proposed concept of death.

References

Andrews, K. (1992), "Managing the persistent vegetative state", *Brit. Med. J.,* vol.305, pp. 486-487.
Aquinas, T. Discussed in Russell, B. (1984), *A History of Western Philosophy,* Unwin, London, p. 449.
Becker, L.C. (1988a), "Human being: the boundaries of the concept", in M.F. Goodman (ed.), *What is a person?,* Humana Press, Clifton, pp. 57-81.
Becker, L.C. (1988b), "Human being: the boundaries of the concept", in M.F. Goodman (ed.), *What is a person?,* Humana Press, Clifton, p. 59.
Beecher, H.K. (1969), "After the 'definition of irreversible coma'", *New Eng. J Med.* vol. 281, pp. 1070-1071.
Davson, H. (1968), in H. Davson and M.G. Eggleton (eds.), *Principles of Human Physiology,* 14th ed., Churchill Livingstone, London, p. 367.
Gervais, K.G. (1986a), *Redefining death.* Yale Univ. Press, New Haven. Gervais, K.G. (1986b), *Redefining death.* Yale Univ. Press, New Haven, p. 52.

Jonas, H. (1974), "Against the stream: comments on the definition and redefinition of death", in H. Jonas, *Philosophical essays: from ancient creed to technological man*, Univ. of Chicago Press, Chicago (reprinted 1980).
Kant, I. *Introduction to logic.* XI, 41, n1. (discussed in Medawar, P. (1984), *The limits of science*, Oxford Univ. Press, London (see above)).
Lamb, D. (1985), *Death, brain death and ethics*, Croom Helm, London.
Lewis, H.E. (1968), in H. Davson and M.G. Eggleton (eds.), *Principles of Human Physiology*, 14th ed., Churchill Livingstone, London, p. 748.
Macknight, A.D.C. (1994), in J.J. Bray, P.A. Cragg, A.D.C. Macknight, R.G. Mills and D.W. Taylor (eds.), *Lecture notes on human physiology*, 3rd ed., Blackwell Science Ltd, Oxford, p. 2.
Medawar, P. (1984), *The limits of science*, Oxford Univ. Press, London.
Nagel, T. (1986), *The view from nowhere*, Oxford Univ. Press, New York, p. 224.
Pallis, C. (1983), *ABC of brainstem death.* Brit. Med. Ass., London, 1983.
Pope Pius XII. (1957), "Prolongation of life", *Pope Speaks*, vol. 4, pp. 393-398.
Popper, K. *Dialectica.* 32:342 (discussed in Medawar, P. (1984), *The limits of science*, Oxford Univ. Press, London. (see above)).
Rachels, J. (1991), *Created from animals. The moral implications of Darwinism*, Oxford Univ. Press, New York, p. 149.
Singer, P. (1988), "All animals are equal", in P. Singer (ed.), *Applied Ethics*, Oxford Univ. Press, New York, p. 215.
Steinbock, B. (1989), "Recovery from persistent vegetative state? The case of Carrie Coons", *Hastings Center Report*, vol. 19(4), pp. 14-15.
Teasdale, G.M and Jennett, B.J. (1974), "Assessment of coma and impaired consciousness: a practical scale", *Lancet*, vol. 2, pp. 81-84.
Veatch, R.M. (1975), "The whole-brain oriented concept of death: an outmoded philosophical formulation", *J. Thanatology*, vol. 3, pp. 13-30. See also Younger, S.J. and Bartlett, E.T. (1983), "Human death and high technology: the failure of the whole-brain formulations", *Ann. Int. Med.*, vol. 99, pp. 252-258.
Veatch, R.M. (1989), *Death, dying and the biological revolution*, Yale Univ. Press, New Haven.
Weissmann, F. (1946), "Language strata", *Synthese*, vol. v, pp. 211-219.

8 Does Anything that Contributes to Homeostasis Count Toward Homeostasis?

"All are but parts of one stupendous whole"
Alexander Pope *An essay on man* Epistle 1, 1.267

Introduction

It should be remembered that I am arguing that death of an organism should be construed as the death of the organism as an integrated whole and not death of the whole organism. I have argued earlier that the concept of death being defended in this monograph is that the permanent loss of the maintenance of bodily integrity constitutes death. The question to be addressed here is whether any component of a system used in homeostasis should have the same value as the control of homeostasis. If I express this question in terms of an abstract system, then the question is whether any component of a system has the same value as the control of the constituent components of the that same system.

Value of System -v- Value of Components of the System

Allow me to examine and explore the differences between the central control of a system and the peripheral components of a system using an abstract/non-biological system in the first instance. In any system with peripheral components contributing to the system and a central area or "black box" exerting control over the system, loss of a peripheral component may, in some circumstances, lead to failure of the system at some later indeterminate time. I have used the phrase "may lead" simply because it is an empirical observation that the loss of some peripheral components in some systems does not invariably lead to failure of the system. For example, it is unlikely that the loss of one single screw from the headlight unit of a car would result in failure of either the headlight unit or the car as a whole, whereas the loss of the bulb would certainly lead to the failure of the headlight unit (although the car would otherwise continue to function normally). In other words, not all components of a given system have the same value to the functioning of the system as a whole. Loss of some components may have little, if any, discernible effect upon the system as a whole and, equally, there are some peripheral components of a system that are necessary for the system to function as such. The question to be addressed here is whether or not any such peripheral component is as important to the system as the central control of the same system. In other words, has a peripheral component of a system the same value to the system as the central control of the same system.

I think that this question can be best explored by the use of an analogy with a steam locomotive. Within any steam locomotive, there are a variety of components *e.g.* boiler, furnace, system of tubes for delivery of steam to the pistons and a controller for the regulation of steam pressure. Each component can function independently of the others to some extent but it is only when the entire collection of components functions as a whole or as a system that we would have a working steam locomotive. Now, with respect to the point explored in the second paragraph concerning the loss of a peripheral component of a system and the effect of such a loss on the system as a whole, it should be obvious that the loss of a peripheral component of a steam locomotive (hereinafter "train") such as a single nut or screw from a protective plate over a wheel for example, would not necessarily lead to interruption or cessation of function of the train as a whole. However, the loss of an increasing number of peripheral components would, eventually, cause the malfunction or complete cessation of function of the train as a whole. In other words, although the loss of one, single peripheral component from the train may not cause failure of that train there is no doubt that continued loss of the peripheral components of the train would result, eventually, in the non-functioning of the train as a train.

I would like to approach this same question from a slightly different angle but using the same analogy. If we consider to the state in which the train is intact but lacks a controller, it is conceivable that some functioning of the train might be produced under these circumstances. However, it is likely that any such functioning would be uncoordinated and ill timed. If we now introduce into the system a functioning controller, we would find that the train would function in a more co-ordinated and normal fashion. It would seem that the addition of a controller to the train results in something that is greater or better than the sum of its parts. Since this higher quality product (normal function of the train) is considered to be the desirable end-point of the components of a train working together, it would seem that the train functions as it is expected to only with the addition of the controller. In terms of an abstract system, it may be possible for the system to function to some degree if the peripheral components are present and functional, but the level and, probably, the complexity, of functioning is raised considerably with the addition of some form of central control. In terms of an abstract system, this set of circumstances would be reproduced if each individual peripheral component was able to function but only in a "free-wheeling" state, *i.e.* functioning totally independently of all the other peripheral components. The addition of a central control to such a system, as in the analogy, would result in the functioning of the peripheral components being co-ordinated; in other words, the system would work as a system as a whole. Hence, in a system in which the peripheral components of the system are totally independent of each other, it is possible that these peripheral components would function correctly (but in an uncoordinated fashion) without any central control. It would require the addition of central control to allow the system to function as a system. In such a system as I have just described, it could be argued that the central control is the "guarantee" that the system will function as a system and not merely as a disjointed and unconnected collection of peripheral components. I will return to this question of "guarantee" later, in order to dismiss it.

It follows from my argument in the previous paragraph that loss of the central control of a system means that the system, as a system, must cease to function at that point. It is, therefore, plain that the loss of a peripheral component of a system is not the same as the loss of the central control of the same system, since in the case of the loss of some of the peripheral components of the system, the system will continue to function whereas in the case of the loss of the central control of the system, the system will cease to function *as a system* immediately. I would now like to return to the analogy of the train and the scenario in which a considerable number of peripheral components have been lost with the result that the train is unable to function as an train. It is, perhaps, not immediately obvious how the non-functioning of the train under these circumstances differs from the non-functioning of the same train after the loss of the controller; it is important that a distinction be made and appreciated. As I have argued already, the loss of the central control unit from a system will result in the immediate loss of the function of that system as a whole. In the case of the loss of a functionally significant number of peripheral components of a system, this loss of the functioning of the system as a system would not be immediate but would occur only after a variable period of time during which the control unit of the system would be attempting to continue to control the system. Only after this variable period of time would the system cease entirely to function as a system. Alternatively, it could be considered that when the central control of a system is lost (*i.e.*, loss of controller within the analogy) the system ceases to function as a system immediately, whereas in the case of a loss of a functionally significant number of peripheral components of the system (*i.e.*, loss of significant numbers of peripheral components within the analogy) the system continues to function as a system, albeit imperfectly, for a variable length of time. Hence the two scenarios envisaged within the analogy, namely loss of function of the train after loss of controller and loss of function of the train after the loss of a functionally significant of peripheral components, are not equivalent but are quite distinct.

In summary, my argument in relation to the non-biological or abstract system that the loss of the central control of the system is not the same as the loss of a peripheral component of the same system can be expressed as follows. Event A (loss of central control) produces outcome Z (loss of normal system function) every time event A occurs and produces it immediately on every occasion. Event B (loss of peripheral component or components of a system) may produce outcome Z or may not produce outcome Z but in neither case does outcome Z occur immediately. The properties of events A and B show no overlap and, therefore, are properties of separate events. In other words, events A and B are separate events. However, one counter-argument against this line of reasoning could use the fact that event B could produce outcome Z immediately if it (*i.e.* event B) is of sufficient magnitude. In this particular set of circumstances, it could be argued that event A and B are equivalent. The argument that events A and B are equivalent rests entirely upon the fact that the same outcome (outcome Z) occurs in both cases. Under the circumstances described, that is event B being so massive that outcome Z is produced immediately, it would be reasonable to consider event A and event B as equivalent in terms of outcome Z since both produce outcome Z immediately. However, it is difficult to conceive of a set of circumstances in biological systems that would allow such equivalence of events A and B in practice. Massive loss of peripheral components of system (e.g. fluid balance) in biological systems is always followed for a variable amount of time by a period of compensation however incomplete, prior to the complete failure of the system involved; this is quite different from the immediate loss of the system when central control has been lost. Therefore, whilst it may be possible to argue that, theoretically, events A and B can be equivalent under some circumstances, this is not the case in practice—the loss of a peripheral component of a biological system is not equivalent to the loss of central control of the same system.

I would now like to return to my previous use of the term "guarantee" and discuss it further. It may be argued here that the control unit of the system (the controller in the analogy) is, in effect, a guarantor that the system will function as a system and could, in some respects, be likened to the guarantee that is acquired with, for example, a car. While the concept of the control unit of a system being considered a guarantor of the functioning of that system is, *prima facie*, an appealing one, I think that the analogy is not one that could, or should, be pursued too far. Let me examine this more closely. Certainly, there are similarities in that in both cases the guarantor and the entity guaranteed are separate physical entities and can exist as such, independently of the other. (I shall return to this question of separate entities later in my discussion relating to biological systems.) However, there are differences that I think are important. In the case of the car and its guarantee, each can exist *as they are* independently of the other and physically separate from the other, but in the case of the controller and the train, this is not the case. In this case, the controller would continue to exist as before but the train would not function as a train in the light of the argument presented earlier. In other words, removal of the guarantor (controller) results in a significant change in the entity being guaranteed such that it no longer exists *as it was*. It is for this reason that I consider that the analogy of the controller being a guarantor is not a useful one. Perhaps it would be more useful to examine again the effect of the controller upon the uncoordinated collection of individual peripheral components that were independent of each other. The effect of the controller was to produce a co-ordinated train that was capable of functioning as such. In terms of abstract systems, the effect of the insertion of the control unit into a collection of individual unconnected peripheral components was to produce a system *that had not existed as a system prior to the insertion of the control unit.* It may be argued from this position that the definition of a system is such that a central control unit is a necessary prerequisite and not merely another contingent peripheral component. If it is the case that a central control unit is a necessary component of a system by definition, it would follow that the loss of such a control unit would result not only in a change in the status of the system from "system" to "collection of uncoordinated peripheral components", but that there would also be a loss of the normal end-product of the system since the uncoordinated activity of the peripheral components could not produce it.

In short, therefore, loss of control of a system results in loss of the system as a system and loss of the normal end products of that system.

I would now like to turn my attention to biological systems and examine the points brought out so far but now in relation to homeostasis in the human being. In an intact human being there are a variety of "systems", for example the cardiovascular, respiratory, endocrine systems each serving its own purpose (Ganong, 1993a). All of these systems have a control mechanism, but some, notably the cardiovascular system, can function within very narrow limits without such control. The problems posed by this continued function of the cardiovascular system (or, more accurately, by the continued function of a component of the cardiovascular system in an imperfect manner) is considered briefly but lucidly by Mason and McCall-Smith (1994). While the normal control mechanism, whatever it may be, functions for any of the systems then the direct comparison is with the train functioning normally under the influence of the controller, the whole system working normally with the normal output. If, however, the control mechanism is removed from any of the biological systems then the comparison is more correctly with the train without the controller; in the biological systems the output would not be "uncoordinated mechanical activity" but an abnormally reduced output (that is, an output that is reduced beyond the normal lower limits for the system) or, in some extreme cases, no output at all. These two states, that is, abnormally reduced output or no output, may not necessarily be immediately detrimental to the whole organism, for example the relative or absolute lack of growth hormone in the human being may not be clinically obvious for many months or years. This happy result is not always the case, however, and immediate loss of respiratory or cardiovascular function would result in death of the human being unless immediate respiratory and cardiovascular support was given.

It should be obvious from the previous discussion that loss of the control mechanism in biological systems will always be detrimental in some way to the human being and in some cases the detriment would be immediate and fatal. Let me now examine the circumstances that would exist if a peripheral component of a biological system ceased to function. As an example let me consider the loss of an area of skin as in a burn. If the area is small, the result would be loss of fluid only; this would be compensated for by the reduction of fluid loss via the kidneys and the extra loss of fluid from the skin, or more correctly from the area of skin loss, would not result in any significant upset to the body as a whole. This state of affairs could correctly be compared to the loss of one or two peripheral components from the train with no noticeable reduction in the functioning of the train. However, it is possible to lose a substantial amount of skin in a burn and it is appropriate that this circumstance be examined. In this case, the loss of fluid would be more severe but, again, compensatory mechanisms would result in reduction of fluid loss from the kidneys even to the extent of no urine output and eventual renal failure. In addition, other compensatory mechanisms would result in constriction of the blood vessels to minimise the effect of fluid loss on the blood pressure and consequently on the blood supply to the organs; this constriction of the blood vessels is performed selectively and blood flow to certain tissues is reduced almost to zero while the supply to other tissues is maintained (Ganong, 1993b). A second effect of the loss of such an area of skin is that the temperature of the affected individual would begin to fall since intact skin is also a peripheral component of the temperature regulating system. This drop in temperature would be compensated for and corrected, completely or incompletely, by elevation of the metabolic rate (that is, the rate of energy production is increased) and constriction of the blood vessels in the periphery of the body (for example, skin); whether these mechanisms would maintain body temperature within normal limits after the loss of a large area of skin would depend upon the area of skin lost and the temperature of the environment, but it is possible that the temperature of the body could be maintained within normal limits indefinitely. These two problems arising from the loss of skin, that is the loss of fluid and loss of heat, would be analogous to the problems produced by the loss of an increasing number of peripheral components by the train. Under these circumstances, the train continues to function but the functioning may not be up to the usual levels and in the case of the biological systems, the organism continues to exist but with some limitation.

    The state of affairs described in the preceding paragraphs illustrate that the loss of the central control unit (whatever that may be) in a biological system is quite a different matter from the loss of one or more of the peripheral components of the same system. However, it could also happen that the loss of one or more of the peripheral components of a biological system could lead to the loss of the control of the system if the compensatory mechanisms are unable to cope with the loss. This loss of control of the system could occur at any time after the loss of the peripheral component, but the important feature under these circumstances is that the loss of control occurs *at some time after* the loss of the peripheral component, whereas the loss of control after loss of the control unit is *immediate*. This difference is analogous to the problems arising with a train that suddenly has the controller removed and a train that has an increasing number of peripheral components removed; in the first instance, the train will stop functioning as a train immediately, and in the second instance the train will stop functioning as a train at some indefinite time in the future. The arguments relating to this have already been laid out in terms of abstract/non-biological systems earlier in this chapter.

So far I have discussed only the problems within a single system in the biological examples, but this is a very oversimplified view of matters. Before I discuss this further in terms of biological systems, it would be useful to examine another scenario within the framework of the analogy. Consider the problems that could potentially arise when two trains must function together, for example in order to move an abnormally heavy load that is beyond the capacity of either train individually. Normally each train will have its own, independent controller when they perform independently, but two independent controllers under these circumstances would not lead to co-ordinated functioning of the two trains. Under these circumstances (that is, joint functioning of two trains), better results would be obtained if the efforts of the two trains were co-ordinated by a single controller. Hence, it may be beneficial to have a single controller controlling, temporarily at least, more than one train. In terms of an abstract system, one controller can, temporarily, exert control over more than one system in order to produce a co-ordinated output.

The question arises as to whether such an arrangement (*i.e.* one single controller with control over more than one system) exists in the biological systems previously discussed in relation to an intact human being. There can be little doubt that this arrangement is represented within normal human biological systems; one has only to read some commonly available texts on human physiology to appreciate quickly that this arrangement is not unusual but is, indeed, the normal state of affairs (Ganong, 1993c). Examples of this integration of biological systems are the response to cold or heat or even the response to such an everyday event as running. This latter activity demands co-ordinated responses from the respiratory, cardiovascular and locomotor systems (not to mention the visual system if obstacles are to be avoided); in addition, if such activity is to be prolonged, then the heat generated by the muscles involved must be lost thus demanding even more integrated activity. This integration and co-ordination of multiple human biological systems illustrates well the concept put forward by Sherrington (1906) that integration is of the greatest importance in the life of a human being. Even if we forget, for the moment, the regulation and integration of these systems that we have been discussing, there are other functions of which the normal human is normally unaware, *e.g.* control of hormone secretion, control of electrolyte balance, control of temperature and control of intestinal activity. All these "systems" are integrated such that they work in a co-ordinated fashion and not, as in the case of the components of a train without a controller, in isolation from each other.

As I have argued in the preceding paragraph, organs working independently of each other would not be sufficient to allow an organism (even one less complex than a human being) to survive and that integration of the organs into a system is necessary for any organism to survive. This argument can be extended and applied to systems instead of individual organs. In order for an organism to survive, the various systems contained within the organism must be controlled individually but, equally importantly, the systems themselves must be co-ordinated in order to produce an appropriate response to a demand from either the environment or the organism itself. This set of circumstances is represented within the analogy by the arrangements described earlier whereby one controller co-ordinated the efforts of both trains with the abnormally heavy load. It is relevant here to bring to mind one important difference between the controller/two trains co-ordination and the systems co-ordination within the human being. In the case of the two trains, both entities are capable of existing without the other and, when separated, regain the appropriate, independent controller. This is not the case in the human being where, if this co-ordination of the systems is lost, the control of the individual, unco-ordinated systems is not sufficient to support the continued existence of the affected human. In order for an organism to survive, it is necessary that this co-ordination function normally; in other words, in biological systems, the "two trains" must always function together in a co-ordinated fashion. I have already argued that the loss of the control of a system is not the same as the loss of a peripheral component of the same system and that in a multiple-system arrangement the co-ordinated control of the multiple systems is equally essential to the overall functioning; it is logical, therefore, to arrive at the conclusion that the loss of multiple system control is not the same as loss of a peripheral component of any of the systems that are being controlled.

The primary question in this chapter has been the one asked at the beginning, *viz.* "Does anything that contributes to homeostasis count toward homeostasis?" and I have presented arguments in the foregoing paragraphs that support my contention that the central control of homeostasis should count toward homeostasis but that the peripheral components should not. A secondary but equally important question that needs to be addressed under the general heading of this section is the rôle of a peripheral component of a system after the system itself has lost its normal control mechanism. If I retain the train analogy that I have used throughout this discussion, the question becomes one about the rôle or status of an individual peripheral component when there is no controller for the train. Under these circumstances, there is no doubt that the peripheral component concerned may continue to function to some extent, but it should be equally clear that this functioning would not be co-ordinated with the functions (if any) of the other peripheral components. In other words, a peripheral component functioning under these conditions would have little, if any, value to the other components of the "system". The value placed upon the peripheral component (or the correct functioning of that peripheral component) is dependent upon the presence of an intact and normally functioning train within which the contribution of the peripheral component normally occurred. In short, therefore, if there is no control over a system there is no system, and if there is no system then the individual contributions from the peripheral components are of little or no value. If we now turn to the human being, we find that the concept of the peripheral components having little or no value in the absence of an intact system is well established. An example would be the attitude to various organs of the body at the time of the death of an individual or soon thereafter. Under the time honoured criteria for establishing death, that is the permanent absence of breathing and the permanent absence of a beating heart, there is no hesitation in pronouncing such an individual dead even although some, if not most, of the cells in that individual's body are still alive; death is the death of the individual and not death of every single cell in that individual. Adoption of this attitude with regard to death implies that no value is placed on these surviving cells and their contribution to what remains of the systems of which they were once a part. In other words, the idea that, in the absence of an intact system, the individual components of that system have little or no value, is one that has been in existence for a considerable time and has been widely adopted both inside and outside medicine, that is adopted by both the medical profession and laymen alike.

What I would like to suggest at this point is that this devaluation of a peripheral component of a system in the absence of an intact system extends to any component of the system. If we devalue one cell under these circumstances we should, logically, also devalue two or more cells under the same circumstances, and in another logical extension, we should devalue any organ (that is any collection of cells) that continues to survive under the same circumstances. This is not a novel suggestion inasmuch as transplant surgeons, at the present time and for some time past, have removed certain organs from human beings who have died using the common criteria of permanent cessation of breathing and heartbeat. In the absence of control of a system, we seem to place no value on the individual components of that system. However, I have argued earlier in this document that overall integration of multiple systems in the human being is of prime importance for the continued existence of the human being, citing Sherrington (1906), and I would now like to extend this idea of the devaluation of cells or an organ to the circumstances that would exist when the co-ordination of the systems has been permanently lost. This must be examined closely because the co-ordination of multiple systems and the control over one individual system are not one and the same thing. Within abstract systems it is easy to conceive of these two ideas, *viz.* loss of overall co-ordination and loss of individual control, as being entirely separate and, indeed, this may be the case in real, non-biological systems. Under these circumstances, it may be possible to argue that the loss of overall co-ordination need not necessarily lead to loss of control of individual systems. In that case, the peripheral components of the individual systems would not be devalued simply because they remain part of the system that retains its own control mechanism despite the loss of overall co-ordination of the multiple systems. Hence, in abstract systems and possibly in some non-biological systems, it would be possible to lose the overall co-ordination of multiple systems but retain the individual control over these systems thereby not devaluing the peripheral components of these systems. This argument could, logically, be used by proponents of the "beating heart" criteria of death to support their view that while integration of a human being has been lost under the circumstances of present-day brain death tests, the beating heart has not been devalued and should still be used as a criterion of death.

Before discussing that particular argument, I would like to continue the more general discussion about the value of the peripheral components of a system when overall integration of the appropriate multiple systems has been lost. I have already explored this question in relation to abstract systems in the previous paragraphs and it is now appropriate that the same question be considered in terms of biological systems and, in particular, in human beings. It is at this point that my earlier *caveat* that the overall co-ordination of multiple systems and the control over one individual system may not be one and the same thing becomes relevant. I have argued earlier that that in abstract systems these two entities are not the same thing either conceptually or in practice, but it is not clear that this particular conclusion can be applied to biological systems. In this latter case, whilst certain concepts and functions can be discussed, and are discussed, separately and in isolation from each other, the reality of the system is such that physical, anatomical or physiological separation of certain functions is not possible. By this I mean that loss of overall co-ordination of multiple systems and loss of control of individual systems will occur together and that loss of one without the simultaneous loss of the other is not possible, once overall co-ordination of the multiple systems has been lost. This indivisible coupling of these two events leads to the conclusion that loss of overall co-ordination of multiple systems is inescapably linked to the loss of control of individual systems and, if my previous arguments are accepted, to inevitable devaluing of any peripheral components that continue to function (however imperfectly). This line of argument would, of course, imply that any individual cells or organs functioning after loss of overall integration of the systems would have little or no functional value, although it may retain a symbolic value. In other words, the beard or finger nails that continue to grow after death (by the conventional or brain death criteria) have no value; this accords closely with present-day beliefs about these post-mortem events as I have discussed earlier in this section. More importantly, however, is the implication of this line of argument for the value of the heart that continues to beat under the circumstances of brain death (by present criteria); if my arguments are accepted, then it follows that the beating heart under these circumstances has little or no functional value. I address this topic of the continued beating of the heart again in greater depth in chapter 10.

I would now like to return to the argument that, although overall control of a system has been lost, local control over one or more of the constituent sub-systems can remain and that this is the state of affairs that exists in relation to the continued beating of the heart in brainstem and whole-brain death. As I pointed out earlier in this chapter, this is a form of argument that could be used by those supporting the "beating heart" criteria of death. While it is true from empirical observation that if all control of the heart from the brainstem and areas above the brainstem are removed, the heart will continue to beat and the heart rate will vary with the volume of blood entering the right atrium of the heart, this does not constitute "control" of the heart and cardiac output in the normal sense of the term "control". This variation in heart rate is a result of a simple stretch reflex initiated in the atrium itself (the Bainbridge reflex) and consists of stretch of the walls of the atrium caused by a greater volume of blood resulting in a greater force of contraction at the next atrial contraction (Davson, 1968). This mechanism cannot alter the cardiac output by any significant amount and is akin to the well-known knee-jerk reflex in which the patellar tendon at the knee is stretched suddenly resulting in the straightening of the knee. To claim that the demonstration of the Bainbridge reflex implies that the heart is still under some form of control is akin to claiming that the demonstration of the knee-jerk implies "control" over the function of the leg or the locomotor system—a claim with no evidence in its support. When the heart continues to beat and vary its rate in brainstem or whole-brain death, there is no logical reason why it should not be viewed in the same way as any other muscle that exhibits a stretch reflex.

Summary

In this section, I have argued that the loss of a peripheral component of a system is not the same as the loss of control of the same system. I have also argued that the overall integration of multiple systems is of more importance than control of an individual system and that loss of overall integration, in biological systems, cannot occur without loss of control of individual systems. Finally, I have argued that the value of the peripheral components of a system is lessened when control of that system is lost and, by extension, is also lessened when overall integration of multiple systems is lost.

References

Davson, H. and Eggleton, M.G. (1968), *Principles of human physiology*, 14th ed., J & A Churchill, London, pp. 210-211.
Ganong, W.F. (1993a), *Review of Medical Physiology*, 16th ed., Appleton & Lange, Connecticut, pp. 469-586, 587-634, 251-425 for examples but whole text is relevant.
Ganong, W.F. (1993b), *Review of Medical Physiology*, 16th ed., Appleton & Lange, Connecticut, pp. 577-581.
Ganong, W.F. (1993c), *Review of Medical Physiology*, 16th ed., Appleton & Lange, Connecticut, pp. 109-252, but especially pp. 208-240.
Mason, K. and McCall-Smith. (1994), *The law and medical ethics*, 4th ed., Butterworths, Edinburgh, pp. 281-282.
Sherrington, C.S. (1906), *The integrative action of the nervous system*, Cambridge Univ. Press, Cambridge, 1906, 1947 (cited in Davson, H. and Eggleton, M.G. (1968), *Principles of human physiology*, 14th ed., J & A Churchill, London, p. 925).

9 Is Brain Death Necessary and Sufficient for Death?

"A man can have but one life and one death"
Robert Browning *In a balcony* 1. 13

Introduction

In earlier chapters, I have put forward arguments supporting my monograph that there are necessary and sufficient conditions for life (chapter 7), that a biological concept of life and death is possible (chapter 8) and that, within this biological concept of life and death, the permanent loss of the control of homeostasis should be considered as the concept of death to be adopted (chapter 8). I must now consider the criteria necessary (in the human being at least) for this suggested concept of death. The organ within which homeostasis is controlled is the brain and, consequently, it is the death of the brain that must now be considered.

Is Brain Death Necessary for Death?

There are two possible meanings to be taken from this question. One of these is "Is it necessary for brain death to be present at the intellectual or philosophical level for death to be considered to exist in any entity?". From the arguments put forward in preceding chapters (chapters 5, 6 and 7 are most pertinent), it is my position that death of an entity could not be considered until the control of homeostasis is permanently lost in that entity. In other words, it is necessary to have permanent loss of homeostatic function before death can occur. Since I have argued that it is necessary to have whole brain death in order to have permanent loss of hypothalamic function, it follows that it is necessary to have whole brain death for death. Other clinical states that involve the permanent non-functioning of large areas of brain and that may appear superficially similar to whole brain death, for example persistent vegetative state and brain stem death (at least in its strict definition), do not encompass this permanent loss of hypothalamic function. It follows, therefore, that whole brain death is necessary for the diagnosis of death.

This conclusion, that is that whole brain death is necessary for the diagnosis of death is reached on the basis of my statement, in the preceding paragraph, that "it is necessary to have whole brain death in order to have permanent loss of hypothalamic function". That statement, however, reflects the *practical* answer to the question posed at the beginning of the second paragraph in this chapter, that is "Is it necessary for brain death to be present at the intellectual or philosophical level for death to be considered to exist in any entity?". At the present level of investigative technology, it is not possible to diagnose hypothalamic death prior to whole brain death occurring, therefore, in practice, whole brain death must be present before hypothalamic death can be ascertained. It should be reiterated here, for the sake of clarity, that hypothalamic death does not occur in the persistent vegetative state, the locked-in syndrome or in brainstem death in its strict interpretation (as I have discussed in chapter 5).

Therefore, I have argued so far that we must consider, *in practice*, that whole brain death is present before we can consider that a human being is dead. However, *intellectually or philosophically*, we are not restricted by the limitations of technology. Under these conditions, whole brain death may not be necessary for death to be considered present in a human being. Let us consider the position in which hypothalamic death can be detected with certainty prior to whole brain death. At this point, we must remember that our prime interest is the permanent loss of control of homeostasis since that is what I advocate as a concept of death. If what we are interested in is the permanent loss of control of homeostasis and we accept that this control resides in the hypothalamus in human beings, then it follows that we are interested in the permanent loss of function of the hypothalamus; the function of the remaining areas of the brain are of no interest to us when we are considering the alive/dead status of an organism. Therefore, intellectually and philosophically, if we are not constrained by the limits of investigative technology, we are necessarily interested in only the permanent loss of function of the hypothalamus and not necessarily in whole brain death when we wish to consider whether or not death has occurred in a human being. Therefore, in answer to the question "Is it necessary for whole brain death to be present at the intellectual or philosophical level for death to be considered to have occurred in a human being?", there are two possible answers:

- if we are restricted to present investigative technology which cannot separate whole brain death and hypothalamic death, then whole brain death is necessary for the diagnosis of death;

- if we are not restricted to present technology and consider a position in which hypothalamic death can be separately (and reliably) detected from whole brain death, then whole brain death is not necessary, but hypothalamic death is necessary, for the diagnosis of death.

It may be argued by those who oppose the idea of a brain-centred concept of death that it is possible to produce death if sufficient destruction of more peripheral areas of the body is caused; under this argument, it would not be necessary to invoke brain death in any of its various forms (including my own) in any concept of death. I have already touched upon this argument in Chapter 8 when I was discussing the possible equivalence of two events, and it is appropriate at this point to return to it but from another direction in order to rebut the argument put forward by the opponents of a brain-centred concept of death. Let us consider, in general terms at present, what happens at the physiological level when an organism is subject to an insult from an external source. The response after such an insult is to minimise the effect such an insult might have on the whole organism, for example avulsion of a limb results in rapid and extreme vasoconstriction to minimise blood loss that could be potentially fatal to the organism. Another example would be the response of an organism to the introduction of foreign protein (for example a virus) which is to raise the temperature of the body; while this is uncomfortable for the organism, it is much more damaging, and usually fatal, to the virus. Such mechanisms have been incorporated into the homeostatic system in the human being. Let us consider what happens if the insult is greater, in fact great enough to present a threat to life (although avulsion of a limb would certainly do that). If the magnitude of the insult is gradually increased, then there will come a point at which any homeostatic mechanism will be overwhelmed and no homeostatic response will occur or, at least, any homeostatic response under these circumstances would be inadequate to return the system disturbed to within normal limits. It would be at this latter point, that is at the point at which the control of homeostasis has been lost, that I would contend that death has occurred. In other words, an insult great enough to produce death, produces death only by overwhelming the homeostatic mechanisms such that control of homeostasis is permanently lost. This rebuttal can be summarised as follows. Insult A produces a disturbance of homeostasis X, such that at some later time the normal homeostatic mechanisms return the disturbed parameters to within normal limits: the organism continues to survive. Insult B produces a disturbance of homeostasis Z, such that the homeostatic mechanisms are unable to return the disturbed parameter to normal and control of homeostasis is permanently lost: the organism dies. My rebuttal of the argument that I suggested may be put forward by those advocating a non-brain-centred concept of death is death occurs when the control of homeostasis is permanently lost and that this is the final common pathway by which all insults to an organism can produce death. If one considers this latter statement for a moment one reaches the conclusion that death has always occurred in this manner, that is the permanent loss of the control of homeostasis, whether or not the medical profession has been able to measure it in these terms or, until recently, even conceive of death in these terms.

The second possible meaning to be taken from the question heading this chapter is "Given that it is accepted that it is necessary for hypothalamic death to exist at a philosophical level for death to exist, is it necessary for hypothalamic death to be established at the practical level before death can be established?". This is quite a different question from the first one but it has important practical consequences. If we accept my argument that death is the permanent loss of the capacity for bodily integration and that the permanent loss of homeostasis is the analogue of this state in the human being, then it follows that the criteria for death within my advocated standards would be the permanent loss of hypothalamic function and the tests for death would be some form of tests for hypothalamic function. However, in many circumstances, there would be practical difficulties in establishing death if hypothalamic function was required to be measured on each and every occasion. (A *reductio* argument here would result in the hypothalamic function of Egyptian mummies being measured!) Fortunately, there are manifestations of death other than those examined in the formal tests of hypothalamic function. The permanent cessation of heartbeat and the permanent cessation of spontaneous breathing have been used for some considerable time as tests for death (see chapter 1) and there is no doubt that a human being demonstrating these signs is dead. It does not matter, for the sake of this argument, whether the permanent loss of these two functions played a role in the aetiology of the permanent loss of hypothalamic function or whether they were a result of it; in both cases the hypothalamus has permanently ceased to function and that state, if my concept of death is accepted, is the criterion for death. I conclude, therefore, that it is not necessary in all cases to establish at a practical level that the hypothalamus has permanently ceased to function by direct tests. However, there is one important caveat to this statement that it is not necessary to establish, at a practical level, that the hypothalamus has permanently ceased to function in all cases in which death is to be determined. The important caveat is that we should be able to deduce that hypothalamic function has permanently ceased in all cases. In other words, if formal tests of hypothalamic function are not being used in the determination of death, then it must be possible from the tests that are being used to deduce that hypothalamic function has permanently ceased. In short, the tests used must either be direct tests of hypothalamic function or indirect tests of hypothalamic function. The permanent cessation of heartbeat and the permanent cessation of breathing are in the group of indirect tests that can be used, and have been used, to detect death. My concept of death encompasses, and puts on a sound philosophical basis, the traditional tests for death. Purists may argue that these indirect tests for death may, theoretically, permit a small period of time to elapse between the permanent cessation of heartbeat and breathing and the permanent loss of hypothalamic function and, as a result, it could be said that death had not occurred at the time of the permanent cessation of heartbeat and breathing but at some other time (in this case a later time). The tests, therefore, would be inaccurate inasmuch as there would be permanent cessation of heartbeat and breathing but no (as yet) permanent loss of control of homeostasis. The answer to this suggestion is twofold:

- Consider the possibility that permanent loss of control of homeostasis has occurred and that heartbeat and breathing are still present—a set of circumstances that occurs in brain death in clinical practice. Under these circumstances, when the heartbeat and breathing cease permanently and are detected as having ceased permanently, the permanent cessation of hypothalamic function has already occurred. Therefore, under these particular circumstances the indirect tests (permanent cessation of heartbeat and breathing) indicate the correct state of affairs.
- Consider the circumstances in which the reverse of the circumstances has occurred, that is there has occurred permanent cessation of heartbeat and breathing leading to permanent loss of hypothalamic function because of hypoxic and hypotensive damage to the hypothalamus. Under these circumstances, there would seem to be a *prima facie* case that the hypothalamus is functioning normally when there is permanent cessation of heartbeat and breathing, that is that the indirect tests for death are inaccurate. However, closer inspection of these circumstances suggests otherwise. Under the circumstances described, that is permanent loss of heartbeat and breathing with intact hypothalamic function, it would need to be established that the cessation of heartbeat and breathing were, indeed, permanent and not

merely temporary phenomena. This establishment of the cessation of the heartbeat and breathing as permanent would require observation of these phenomena over some time. During this observation time, the hypotension and hypoxia necessarily induced by the cessation of heartbeat and breathing would produce permanent damage in the hypothalamus (and at other sites within the brain) resulting, in turn, in permanent cessation of hypothalamic function. Therefore, at the point in time at which it can be said that there has occurred permanent cessation of heartbeat and breathing, permanent damage has occurred to the hypothalamus resulting in permanent loss of hypothalamic function. Hence, under the circumstances being discussed (permanent cessation of heartbeat and breathing prior to permanent loss of hypothalamic function), the indirect tests for death, that is the permanent cessation of heartbeat and breathing, would not, in practice, produce an inaccurate result.

In summary, therefore, it is reasonable to say that the indirect tests for death, that is the permanent cessation of heartbeat and breathing, would accurately reflect the permanent cessation of hypothalamic function under all practical circumstances; there would be no false positive or false negative results. It should be noted here that hypoxia (however caused) severe enough and prolonged enough to produce permanent loss of hypothalamic function would also produce, in practice, permanent loss of function of the whole brain. In other words, hypoxia that produces permanent loss of hypothalamic function will also produce whole brain death.

I repeat my earlier conclusion—that it is not necessary in all cases to establish by direct tests at a practical level that the hypothalamus has ceased to function in order to diagnose death if my suggested concept of death is adopted.

Is Brain Death Sufficient for Death?

I have argued in an earlier section on "Can there be necessary and sufficient conditions for life?" (chapter 6) that the basic properties of all living entities were well summarised by Schrödinger (1944). These properties consist of the ability to maintain a low entropy state despite a variety of external entropy states (by external, I mean external to the living entity under consideration). While this property is most easily seen and understood in single-cell organisms, the property is possessed by all living entities. In the human being, this property of maintaining a low entropy state is demonstrated by the ability to maintain homeostasis, that is the ability to maintain a constant internal environment despite changes in the external environment. I have also argued that this capacity for homeostasis is the logical criterion for death if it be accepted that death is the permanent loss of the ability to maintain bodily integrity (in Schrödinger's terms, the permanent loss of the ability to maintain a low entropy state).

The question now becomes one of establishing where this capacity for homeostasis resides in an intact human being. This is a relatively straightforward question to answer inasmuch as physiologists have demonstrated the fact that the hypothalamus in the human brain is responsible for the control of homeostasis, and that damage to a variety of areas within the hypothalamus results in imperfect control or loss of control of some of the facets of homeostasis. From such evidence, it is reasonable to deduce that the capacity for homeostasis resides in the hypothalamus. It follows from the preceding argument that permanent loss of function of the hypothalamus would result in permanent loss of homeostasis.

Now, I have already argued that permanent loss of homeostasis results in the entity concerned undergoing change in ontological status from "alive" to "dead" (see chapters 6 and 7), and it remains for me to consider the clinical conditions in which the functions of the hypothalamus are permanently lost. From the clinical point of view, the condition of whole brain death produces permanent loss of hypothalamic function. It would seem, therefore, from a combination of argument, physiological data and clinical observation, that one condition sufficient to produce permanent loss of hypothalamic function is whole brain death. Whole brain death is, therefore, sufficient for the diagnosis of death if the concept of death that I am advocating is adopted since nothing other than the permanent loss of control of homeostasis is required for death and this requirement is satisfied by the concept of whole brain death. Strictly speaking, the preceding argument that whole brain death is a sufficient condition for death whilst true is over-sufficient and not specific. The statement that that the permanent loss of control of homeostasis is supplied by the permanent loss of hypothalamic function leads only to the conclusion that the permanent loss of hypothalamic function (that is hypothalamic death) is a sufficient condition for death. This is the logically correct deduction from the given premises. The next step, that is from arguing that the permanent loss of function of the hypothalamus is sufficient for death if death is accepted as the permanent loss of control of homeostasis to arguing that whole brain death is a sufficient condition for death, is a step forced upon me by practical considerations. As I have stated earlier in this chapter, it is simply not possible with current investigative technology to detect the permanent loss of hypothalamic function prior to the occurrence of whole brain death as measured by current standards and tests. Whilst, therefore, I have argued that permanent loss of hypothalamic function is a sufficient condition for death, in practice I must accept that whole brain death is a sufficient condition for death if death is accepted as the permanent loss of control of homeostasis.

However, those who oppose the idea of a brain-centred concept of death may suggest that while brain death is necessary for death and is predictive of death, it is not sufficient for death. Indeed, this view has been taken in the past (Conference, 1976) by those who strongly question brain death as death at present (Conference, 1979). Such a group, ably led by Jonas (1974) and Evans (1990), would argue that death has occurred, under these circumstances, only when the heart has stopped beating. At this point we must examine the basis of the selection of the heart as one of the two organs of choice for the determination of death under the traditional criteria for death. There are many organs and organ systems in the body that must function normally in order that the organism as a whole continues to function. However, many of the functions of many of the organs and organ systems are not easily or readily detectable (and some are yet to be established) and the most obvious signs of functioning of the major organ systems of the body are the movement of the chest caused by breathing and the palpable pulse caused by the beating heart (see Chapter 1 for further discussion of the variety of tests for death). Historically, these signs may well have been chosen simply because they could be detected and had an adequate predictive value for death. Under normal circumstances, this choice of tests for death is satisfactory. However, we are not discussing "normal circumstances", and it is appropriate, therefore, that we examine the signs being suggested by the opponents of a brain-centred concept of death. In the absence of breathing and assisted ventilation and in the presence of the permanent loss of the control of bodily integrity, the rôle and significance of the continued beating of the heart should be examined. Under these circumstances, the rate of the beating heart is unusually low with a very low volume of blood pumped out with each beat. In other words, the heart although beating is not capable of providing an adequate circulation to the organs. Will this state of affairs change if the human being under these circumstances is mechanically ventilated? Under these latter circumstances, the blood being moved, albeit imperfectly, by the beating heart contains oxygen and will to some extent provide oxygen to the tissues reached by the blood. This is the only difference between the two circumstances. In both sets of circumstances, the heart is beating simply because of the intrinsic property of cardiac muscle for spontaneous contraction; there is no control over the heart in terms of heart rate, blood pressure or cardiac output. The continued beating of the heart, under these circumstances, can be likened to the continued growth of nails and hair that occurs after death (by normal, conventional criteria). The continued growth of the nails and hair are not taken as signs of continued life of the human being as a whole but merely manifestations of a greater tolerance to low oxygen levels by the tissues concerned compared to other tissues in the body. Similarly, the continued beating of the heart under the conditions of permanent loss of control of bodily integrity and independently of whether or not the human being is being mechanically ventilated is merely a manifestation of the intrinsic properties of cardiac muscle and not a sign of continued life of the human being as a whole. Evans has argued cogently that whole brain death is not sufficient for death but that the inclusion of some form of cardiac criteria is necessary (Evans, 1994a). In his argument against those who advocate a brain-centred concept of death, Evans suggests that

> "together with the rise and fall of the chest, it is the perfusion of the body with blood that offers the clearest visible sign of life in an otherwise motionless and unconscious individual. Our attitude to someone that we see as alive is fundamentally different from our attitude to someone we see as dead. The relevant difference is plausibly charted by the change from a pink, warm and perfused individual to a cold, grey, non-perfused body." (Evans, 1994b)

What am I to make of this argument that:
- whole brain death is not sufficient for death and cardiac criteria need to be included;
- a warm, pink perfused body is alive but a cold, grey non-perfused body is not alive;
- the "clearest visible sign of life" should be taken as the sufficient condition for life.

To some extent I have provided an answer to the first part of Evans' argument in the immediately preceding paragraph. Heart muscle continually contracts because this is one of the physiological properties of heart muscle and it will continue to contract even in the absence of blood in the chambers of the heart. If a human being becomes exsanguinated from extreme loss of blood, the heart would continue to beat although detection of the heartbeat may be very difficult using everyday conventional techniques. Under these circumstances, the human being would not match the description given by Evans (1994b), that is the human being would have a beating heart but would not be pink, warm or perfused—a human being in such circumstances would be cold, grey and non-perfused, while the heart was still beating. What would those who support the beating heart/breathing criteria for death say under these circumstances? Evans would have to choose between saying:

- such a human being is alive because of the persistent heartbeat;
- such a human being is not alive because they are not pink, warm and perfused.

I suspect that Evans would reject the second option and argue that, although pink, warm and perfused means that a human being is alive, the converse does not apply, that is a cold, grey non-perfused human being is not necessarily dead in all cases. The conclusion from this is that it seems that the "warm, pink perfused" criteria is not of prime importance but that we must search for a heartbeat. Evans (1990), like Jonas (1974) suggests that the heartbeat "counts for life", whilst saying that human life does not essentially consist in the heartbeat; the spontaneously persistent heartbeat is to be taken as a sign that the individual concerned is not dead. Evans challenges "those who would exclude the spontaneously persistent heartbeat from counting for life must convince us of their case" (Evans, 1990). I will try since I must do so to argue that brain death is a sufficient condition for death.

Let us consider a human being who has just satisfied my suggested criteria for death, that is permanent loss of control of homeostasis, manifest by permanent loss of hypothalamic function. The heart in such an individual will continue to beat for some hours although that individual will gradually become colder and less pink. In addition, such an individual will become less perfused as the effects of hypoxia or anoxia (from lack of breathing or ventilation) affect the heart muscle. Eventually, there comes a time when there will be no detectable output from the heart, then (a little later) no detectable heart beat by auscultation and then, finally, no detectable cardiac muscle activity as measured electrocardiographically (that is, by ECG). It is not clear to me at which point along this spectrum of cardiac activity those who advocate the beating heart as a criterion for life and death decisions would wish to say that there was no heartbeat. Conventionally, at present, the lack of a heartbeat would be declared when it was not possible to hear the heartbeat by auscultation. However, for some indeterminate time prior to this, there would be no output from the failing, weakening heart. Therefore, during this time that there was a beating heart detectable by auscultation but no cardiac output, the heart muscle would be contracting to no effect—just "twitching". Is the nominal status of an individual in terms of dead or alive to depend upon the presence or absence of a "twitching" muscle? I would suggest that the answer to that question should be "No" and that to answer otherwise is to adopt a stance that is very difficult to defend. Life consists of much more than a "twitching" muscle especially when it is borne in mind that the same piece of muscle would twitch identically if it were placed, extracorporeally, in a nutrient solution and left alone. Life, I contend, consists of the integration of an individual (human or non-human) and not merely in the ineffectual, partial functioning of one of that individual's organs.

Another line of attack against those who hold that the beating heart is important in the determination of life and death in all cases is to enquire of those who hold such a position, what the precise criteria are and when these criteria have been satisfied (I have touched upon the difficulties in the preceding paragraph); when this has been answered, it should then be asked from whence these criteria came. By this I mean what concept of death gives rise to the criteria of breathing and the beating heart. I have discussed the present concepts of death in chapter 4 and the criteria of the beating heart and breathing would seem to be most easily accommodated by the concept of death that holds that death has occurred when there has been "irreversible loss of the flow of vital fluids". The objection to this concept of death that I raised in chapter 4 merits repetition here. This "flow of vital fluids" is merely a manifestation of a complex collection of organic systems and subsystems and is normally controlled within narrow limits by these systems; the essentially important feature is not the flow of fluids however vital they may be, but the control exerted over the flow as part of an integrated whole organism.

From these arguments, it is my contention that whole brain death is sufficient for the diagnosis of death and that the persistence of the beating of the heart under these circumstances has no significance in the determination of whether or not a human being is dead or alive.

Summary

I have presented arguments to support my contention that whole brain death is both necessary and sufficient for the diagnosis of death, but that it is not necessary in all cases of death to establish directly, in practice, the permanent loss of homeostatic function. In practice in the majority of cases, as I have argued, it is necessary only to infer or deduce that the permanent loss of hypothalamic function has occurred, using indirect evidence, *i.e.* by traditional cardio-respiratory means. I have also argued that, under the conditions of permanent loss of homeostasis, the continued beating of the heart has no significance in the determination of death.

References

Conference of the Royal Medical Colleges and their Faculties in the United Kingdom, (1976), "Diagnosis of Brain Death", *Brit. Med. J.*, vol. 2, p. 1187.

Conference of the Royal Medical Colleges and their Faculties in the United Kingdom, (1979), "Diagnosis of Brain Death", *Brit. Med. J.*, vol. 1, p. 332.

Evans, M. (1990), "A plea for the heart", *Bioethics,* vol. 4(3), pp. 227-231.

Evans, M. (1994), "Against the definition of brainstem death", in R. Lee and D. Morgan (eds), *Death Rites,* Routledge, London, p. 6.

Jonas, H. (1974), "Against the stream: comments on the definition and re-definition of death", in *Philosophical Essays,* Prentice-Hall, New Jersey, pp. 132-140.

Schrödinger, E. (1944), *What is life?,* Cambridge Univ. Press, Cambridge, (reprint 1992), pp. 67-75.

10 When does Death Occur?

"Do not go gently into that good night,
Old age should burn and rave at close of day;
Rage, rage against the dying of the light"
Dylan Thomas *Do Not Go Gentle into that Good Night.* v. 1

Introduction

I have already argued that the permanent loss of the ability to maintain bodily integrity entails death and that, in the human being at least, the criterion for this would be the permanent loss of control of homeostasis (see chapter 6) and if that is to be accepted then I must consider the point at which death occurs conceptually. It is of some importance to stress, at the beginning of this discussion, that the topic being addressed is the time at which death occurs conceptually and not the point at which death can be said to have occurred in practice. This latter point in time is quite a separate issue and will be discussed later in this chapter. It is appropriate at this point to repeat that the concept of death that is proposed and defended in this monograph is that "the irreversible loss of function of the organism as a whole", *i.e.* the death of the organism as an integrated whole and not the death of the whole organism. Without the ability to maintain bodily integrity, an entity is unable to maintain other functions including those functions that may be considered unique to it—for example a human being without the ability to maintain bodily integrity would not be able to maintain consciousness or any other function dependent upon consciousness. In other words, the ability to maintain bodily integrity is the base upon which other "higher" functions are dependent and is common to all living entities. There are three obvious candidates for the point at which death can be said to have occurred conceptually:
- at the point at which the whole organism fails;
- at the moment of the lethal insult to the control of homeostasis;
- at the moment of the manifestations of the loss of control of homeostasis.

I shall discuss these in turn.

At the Point at which the Whole Organism Fails

Prior to discussion about the possible selection of this point as the time at which death of an organism occurs conceptually, it is necessary to discuss the possible meanings of the phrase "at the point of failure of the whole organism". There are a variety of possible meanings:
- at the point of failure to work as an integrated functioning unit;
- at the point of wholesale failure in terms of cessation of function throughout its many parts;
- at the point of its material destruction.

These three meanings are not mutually exclusive and it is possible to conceive of a set of circumstances in which all three are simultaneously satisfied, for example in physical destruction of an organism in close proximity to a large explosion. The third meaning, that is "at the point of its material destruction" is rare in practice and need not be considered separately since if the third has occurred, the first and second have also occurred. The two meanings that require most discussion are the first and second.

At the point of failure to work as an integrated functioning unit. The important word in this interpretation of the phrase "at the point of failure of the whole organism" is the word "integrated". Inclusion of this term implies that integration of functions is more important than mere presence of the same functions. This is a point that I have argued already in chapter 8, in which I presented the argument that homeostasis can be controlled only in the presence of integration of the various functions that are required for such control and that the functions *per se* while necessary for the control of homeostasis are not sufficient. If my monograph that permanent loss of control of homeostasis entails death is adopted and my point that control of homeostasis requires the various functions to be integrated is accepted, then it seems tautological to state that death occurs conceptually when this integration of functions is lost. In other words, to state that death occurs conceptually "at the point of failure to work as an integrated functioning unit" is true but does not answer or extend or enhance our understanding of the original question "When does death occur conceptually?". While this answer is a form of answer, I would suggest that it is not the answer that is required and that another answer should be sought.

At the point of wholesale failure in terms of cessation of function throughout its many parts. This is another possible meaning of the phrase "at the point at which the whole organism fails". We must now explore what this means in practice. In practical terms, the phrase implies that all the parts or organs of an organism have ceased to function. If we assume that this cessation of function of all the organs of an organism is permanent and irreversible, then I would suggest that an organism satisfying such a criterion should be viewed as dead. I cannot conceive of a form of argument that would convince me that an organism satisfying the criterion of permanent and irreversible loss of function of all its constituent parts or organs could be viewed as being in any state other than dead. While it is tempting to equate this state with the clinical state of permanent and irreversible cessation of heartbeat and breathing, this would not be correct. At the point of permanent and irreversible cessation of heartbeat and breathing and for a short time afterward, other parts or organs of a human being continue to function, for example nails and hair continue to grow, and muscle cells will continue to contract although for a shorter time than the nails and hair continue to grow. It is obvious, therefore, that the point of permanent and irreversible cessation of heartbeat and breathing is not the same point as the point of the permanent and irreversible cessation of function of all the constituent parts or organs of an organism, although this latter state will be reached at some indefinite time after the former state has been reached.

There is also the temptation to equate the permanent and irreversible cessation of function of the parts or organs of an organism with the condition of putrefaction. Whilst suggestions that this condition should be used as an indicator of when death has occurred have been made (see chapter 1), it should be appreciated that such suggestions were made in the context of ascertaining when death had occurred in practice, not when death had occurred conceptually. I am concerned, here, with the point at which death occurs conceptually and while it is true that putrefaction is a process that occurs only in dead tissue, it is also true that the tissue concerned must be dead prior to the process of putrefaction taking place. Therefore, death has occurred prior to putrefaction and the presence of putrefaction can only indicate that the tissue affected is already dead and has been dead for an unknown time. Putrefaction cannot, therefore, be used either as a reliable indicator of when death occurred in practice or as an indicator of when death occurred conceptually although it may be used to indicate that death of tissues has occurred at some earlier time. Indeed, putrefaction, *per se*, cannot even be used to indicate reliably the death of the organism. Let me expand on that statement. I have made reference, up till now, to the presence of putrefaction in tissues but this only indicates death of the affected tissues. It should be remembered that isolated putrefaction may occur in well-circumscribed tissues of an organism, with the remainder of the organism being apparently normal. An example of this is gangrene and putrefaction in the lower limb of a human being with peripheral vascular disease. In this example, two relevant facts are not in question:

- there is putrefaction;
- the individual so affected is still alive, albeit unwell.

It would seem, therefore, that the presence of putrefaction, *per se*, while sufficient for the diagnosis of death of some of the tissues within the organism, is not sufficient for the diagnosis of death of an organism. Certainly, it may be argued (correctly in my opinion) that an organism that has a sufficient number of its parts or organs affected by putrefaction will die. However, this requires our statement about putrefaction to be modified in some way—specification of site affected and/or number of organs affected—and does not count against my argument that putrefaction *per se* is not a reliable indicator of the death of the organism. The presence of putrefaction even affecting the whole organism is not necessary for the diagnosis of death of the same organism. Consider the position with the mummified Egyptian remains. These remains have never displayed putrefaction—the process of mummification was designed to prevent it— and yet there can be no doubt that the human being in question is dead. Therefore, the presence of putrefaction is not necessary for the diagnosis of death. Hence, putrefaction *per se* is neither sufficient nor necessary for the diagnosis of death, although it can be used as a reliable indicator of the permanent and irreversible cessation of function of parts of an organism. Since putrefaction *per se* is neither necessary nor sufficient for the diagnosis of death, it follows from my previous argument (in the first paragraph of this section) that the permanent and irreversible cessation of function of the parts or organs of an organism indicates the death of the organism that putrefaction cannot be equated with this state of permanent and irreversible cessation of function of the parts or organs of an organism.

Having discussed the rôle of putrefaction in the determination of the point of death conceptually in relation to the permanent and irreversible loss of function of all its constituent parts, I would like to return to the discussion of the relationship between the permanent and irreversible cessation of heartbeat and breathing and the permanent and irreversible loss of function of all the constituent parts of an organism. I have already argued that it would be erroneous to equate the permanent and irreversible cessation of heartbeat and breathing with the permanent and irreversible cessation of function of all the parts and organs in an organism. However, an organism in which there has occurred a permanent and irreversible cessation of heartbeat and breathing is generally considered to be dead. If, therefore, there is a state (namely, permanent and irreversible cessation of heartbeat and breathing) that is considered to entail death and, at the same time, other parts and organs of that same organism are functioning, it should be clear that such time at which there occurs the permanent and irreversible cessation of function of all the parts and organs of an organism cannot represent the time at which death can be considered to have occurred either for practical purposes or, more importantly, in conceptual terms. We should be clear at this point that the permanent cessation of function of all parts and organs of an organism indicates that the organism is dead (or that death has occurred) but cannot be used as a criterion to indicate the time at which death occurred for either practical or conceptual purposes.

At the Moment of the Lethal Insult to the Control of Homeostasis

If the point at which death occurs conceptually (if it is accepted that the permanent loss of control of homeostasis entails death) is not to be taken as the point of failure of the whole organism, but to be taken as some earlier time, then the moment of the lethal insult to the control of homeostasis seems a reasonable candidate for discussion. Indeed, there seems to be a strong *prima facie* case for this suggestion, especially since the use of the term "lethal" appears, modifying the severity of the insult. It would seem that if the insult to the control of homeostasis is severe enough to be referred to as "lethal" then there can be little doubt that this point is the point at which death occurred almost by definition. However, there is a problem with this argument and it hinges on the term "lethal" which is commonly defined as "able to cause or causing death". This implies that an insult referred to as "lethal" is capable of causing death immediately or, importantly, of causing death at some later time in the immediately foreseeable future. Lethal injuries causing death immediately would be events such as decapitation or physical destruction as a result of an explosion, but other injuries less severe than this could also be referred to as "lethal" because death will ensue in the immediate future. In this latter case, the term is being used not to imply that death has occurred but to imply that death will inevitably and directly result. In other words, the term "lethal" is being used as a predictive and causal term. It should be obvious that if the term "lethal" is being used with this predictive meaning then the point of death is not at the point of the lethal insult but at some later time. Within this interpretation of the term "lethal", therefore, the time that death occurs conceptually cannot be the moment of the lethal insult to the control of homeostasis.

If we restrict ourselves, therefore, to the circumstances in which the term "lethal" is being applied to insults that result in the instantaneous and permanent loss of control of homeostasis, then I would suggest that a problem still remains in accepting this as the point at which death occurs. This problem, I should stress, is entirely a practical one. If the control of homeostasis is lost at the point of the insult, there can be no way in which it can be known at that point in time (that is simultaneous with the injury) whether this loss is temporary or permanent. If the loss of control of homeostasis is merely temporary, then the requirement for death in terms of my monograph has not been satisfied. The majority of insults in clinical medicine are of this type, that is it cannot be determined immediately if the insult has been lethal or not. It can be seen, therefore, that it would be unsafe to adopt this point as the point of death *in practice* despite the moment of the lethal insult to the control of homeostasis (when the control of homeostasis is immediate and permanently lost) being the time at which death occurred *conceptually* in such cases.

At the Moment of the Manifestations of the Loss of Control of Homeostasis

I have argued in a preceding section that the point at which there is permanent and irreversible cessation of function of all the parts and organs of the organism cannot be the point at which death occurs conceptually if we accept my monograph that the permanent loss of control of homeostasis entails death. Furthermore, it was explicit in my argument that this latter point had occurred prior to the former point, that is death had occurred conceptually prior to the time at which there was a permanent and irreversible cessation of function of all the parts and organs of the organism. I will now discuss a point in time that occurs earlier than the permanent and irreversible cessation of function of all parts and organs of an organism, namely the point at which the manifestations of the permanent loss of control of homeostasis are apparent or can be detected and assess whether or not this could be the point at which death occurs conceptually if my monograph is adopted.

There is possible ambiguity in the phrase "at the moment of the manifestations of the loss of the control of homeostasis" and clarification is needed prior to further discussion in this section. The phrase could mean either:

- the time *at* which it can be truly said that a permanent loss of control of homeostasis has occurred (time (a));

or

- the time *of* which it can be truly said that a permanent loss of control of homeostasis has occurred (time b)).

Clearly the second may predate first, but not the reverse; at any rate, the two possible meanings are not identical.

The Time at Which It Can Be Truly Said that a Permanent Loss of Control of Homeostasis has Occurred

The point at which it can be truly said that a permanent loss of control of homeostasis has occurred is the point at which investigations and tests are capable of detecting the changes that have occurred as a result of the permanent loss of control of homeostasis. Since these changes take a variable amount of time to reach a level detectable by current investigations, the time at which a positive detection occurs will always postdate the permanent loss of control of homeostasis that produced the changes that were detected. Hence time (b) may predate time (a) but not the reverse. Although it may be argued from the above discussion that time (b) *must* predate time (a), I have only stated that time (b) *may* predate time (a) simply because there are exceptional circumstances in which time (a) and time (b) occur simultaneously, for example when an organism is physically destroyed instantly in an explosion. Under this particular set of circumstances, time (a) and time (b) will occur at the same moment. However, this does not affect the assertion that time (a) can never predate time (b) and under most circumstances time (b) will predate time (a). Therefore, the point at which it can be truly said that a permanent loss of control of homeostasis has occurred is not the point at which the permanent loss of control of homeostasis actually occurred but merely the point at which it can be detected. If more sensitive tests are devised that allow more subtle changes to be detected, then the time at which it can be truly said that permanent loss of control of homeostasis has occurred (that is the time at which the changes consequent upon the loss of control can be detected) will move closer to the time at which the changes began (that is the time at which the loss actually occurred as opposed to the time at which the changes can be detected). It is unlikely, on practical grounds, however, that these two distinct times will ever coincide or merge, that is time (a) will become time (b), except in the case of an explosion as discussed earlier in this section.

Time (a) represents merely the point at which changes consequent upon the permanent loss of control of homeostasis can be detected and can be used to allow it to be truly said that the relevant event has occurred; it does not allow the time at which the event actually occurred to be assessed. In other words, time (a) the moment at which we can truly say that a permanent loss of control of homeostasis has occurred is not the time when death has occurred conceptually if we accept my monograph that the permanent loss of control of homeostasis entails death.

The Time of Which It Can Be Truly Said that Loss of Control of Homeostasis has Occurred

This phrase is one possible meaning of the phrase used earlier in section (iii), namely "at the manifestation of the loss of control of homeostasis" and I have discussed the alternative meaning in the immediately preceding paragraphs. The point under discussion at present is the point at which there occurs conceptually a loss of control of homeostasis and this point needs to be distinguished clearly from the point at which this loss of control of homeostasis can be detected. An analogy may help to separate the two points. Consider a pathologist examining a dead body and consider that:
- the pathologist is the first medically qualified person to examine it;
- the time of death is required for legal purposes.

Now, from this examination of the body he can say that the body is dead (that is, the time *at* which it can be said that the body is dead) at the time of the examination and from further examination he can ascertain that death has occurred some hours or days earlier (the exact time interval is irrelevant to this argument) prior to his examination (that is, the time *of* which it can be said that death has occurred). The point to be taken from this is that there is a time *at* which it could be said that the person was dead and a separate and earlier time *of* which it could be said that death had occurred. Allow me to return to the discussion in which I argued that the point at which permanent loss of control of homeostasis could be said to have occurred was the point at which the manifestations of this loss of control could be measured by physiological or biochemical tests and, as this point was dependent upon the sophistication of the technology employed in the detection process, it may move closer to or further away from the time at which the control of homeostasis had been lost. It is the nature of a physiological process such as homeostasis that when it ceases to function changes occur and that these changes, at the beginning, are small but become greater with time. However, the point at which at which the particular process ceased to function is the point of which it can be said that the process ceased to function although detection of the cessation of function is not possible until some time later. In other words, there is a point when we think of, or conceive of, a function ceasing although we cannot detect the changes consequent upon that cessation of function until some time later and, therefore, have no evidence of the cessation of function. The conceptual time of loss of function is the time of which it can be said that the loss of function occurred. If we use this line of argument in relation to the loss of control of homeostasis, the time of which it can be said that the permanent loss of control of homeostasis has occurred is the point that we conceive of the control of homeostasis being lost although detection of the loss of control will not (or cannot for practical purposes) occur until later. If that is the case, then the point at which death occurs in terms of my monograph that permanent loss of control of homeostasis entails death is the point of which it can be said that permanent loss of control of homeostasis has occurred. All other, later points are points at which death can be said to have occurred already.

This could be illustrated by using the analogy with the train that I used in chapter 8. Consider a train moving at speed (the exact speed is unimportant and irrelevant) along a straight track with all its components and controller intact. The equivalent question, within the analogy, to the question "When does death occur?" would be "When does the train stop functioning as a train?". I have argued that the answer to this question is that death occurs at the point when there is no longer an integrated whole organism and that death is the point of which it can be said that the permanent loss of control of homeostasis has occurred. This point would occur, in the analogy, if the controller stopped working permanently. At first, there would be no evidence of this loss of controller but the train would, inevitably and imperceptibly at first, begin to slow down. At some later point the train would be moving at a speed at which it would be appreciated that, whilst the boiler and other components were all present, there was no co-ordinated activity and the controller was permanently non-functioning. This point of appreciation of these facts would be analogous to the point at which it could be truly said that a permanent loss of control of homeostasis had occurred and is obviously later than the time of which it can be truly said that the permanent loss of control of homeostasis has occurred. Eventually the train will come to complete halt once its kinetic energy has been expended. It would be very easy to equate this point with "the point of wholesale failure in terms of cessation of function throughout its many parts" but I do not think that such equivalence is correct. When the train finally ceases to move, some components may continue to function for a little longer, *e.g.* there may still be some power left to keep lights working. Therefore, some parts of the train may continue to function for a short time; this would be akin to the continued growth of finger nails and beard after the death of a human being. The point of wholesale failure in terms of cessation throughout its many parts would arrive when all functions of the different systems of the train have ceased to function, *i.e.* no lights, no steam or any other function. Eventually, if left alone, it would rust and it would become obvious that the train had not functioned for some time; this point in time would be analogous to the discovery of putrefaction in a human being. In both cases, if the rust or putrefaction affects enough of the train or human being respectively, then there would be no doubt that the train or human being has ceased to function but, importantly, it would also be apparent that this cessation of function had occurred at some earlier time. It should also be obvious that rust could affect the train while it is still functioning normally (with an intact controller)—a small amount of rust on a wheel cover, for example, would not impede or reduce the function of the train. This is analogous to the appearance of putrefaction in an ischaemic lower limb of a human being— putrefaction is undoubtedly present but the affected human being is also undoubtedly alive.

The analogy with the train illustrates well the arguments that I have presented in this chapter but also illustrates the problems with the beating heart/breathing criteria for death. In the analogy with the train, the beating heart and breathing would be represented by the furnace (breathing) and the boiler and the movement of the steam to the pistons (beating heart). When the train is moving forward as described in the previous paragraph and the controller is permanently disconnected, the furnace will cool (if we assume that the furnace had an automatic feed under the controller and would, therefore, be deprived of fuel when the controller was disconnected) and consequently the pressure in the boiler and tubes leading to the pistons will fall, eventually to zero. The cold furnace and zero pressure in the steam system would be analogous, *prima facie*, to cessation of heartbeat and breathing. However, the train may not have stopped at that point in time since its kinetic energy (momentum) may allow it to travel some distance before stopping and the furnace may be cold with zero steam pressure prior to any cessation of movement of the train. There would also be a point in time when there would be some steam in the system but insufficient to produce movement of the pistons. What point, then, is analogous to the permanent cessation of heartbeat and breathing—the cold furnace/zero steam pressure, cessation of movement of the train or some earlier time when the steam pressure is insufficient to produce piston movement (and, therefore, movement of the train)? I have discussed in greater depth the problem of the point that could plausibly be taken as death by supporters of the beating heart/breathing criteria in chapter 9 and I do not intend to pursue it further here; the use of the analogy with the train illustrates well the dilemma discussed in chapter 9.

Summary

In this chapter, I have argued that if my monograph that the permanent loss of control of homeostasis entails death is accepted then the point at which death occurs conceptually is the time of which it can be said that permanent loss of control of homeostasis has occurred. I have also presented arguments to the effect that this time is not the same as the time at which the clinical, physiological or biochemical manifestations of the permanent loss of control of homeostasis can be detected. Whilst this time is conceptually the same time as the time of the lethal insult to the control of homeostasis, it would be unsafe to adopt this point as the point of death in practice.

11 Operational Changes as a Result of the Suggested Concept of Death

"Tempora mutantur, et nos mutamur in illis"
("Times change, and we change with them")
Anon

Introduction

The concept of death that I have put forward in this monograph, *i.e.* that death of an organism as a whole is entailed by the irreversible loss of control of bodily integrity, is not obviously related to either the current brain stem death concept of death or the more commonly used beating heart/breathing criteria, although I have already argued in chapter 9 that the beating heart/breathing criteria could be derived from the concept of death that I advocate. I propose, in this chapter, to discuss the changes in the practice of reaching the diagnosis of death that would necessarily accrue should the suggested concept of death be adopted. It is necessary, before discussing any operational changes in the diagnosis of death, to consider the criteria and tests that are in use under the present concepts of death. At present in the UK there are two separate sets of criteria for the diagnosis of death:
- cardio-respiratory criteria;
- brainstem death criteria.

I intend to examine these criteria and the associated tests prior to examining the criteria and tests that would be logically derived from my suggested concept of death.

Cardio-respiratory Criteria

These criteria are the most widely used in the UK and elsewhere. The criteria state that any individual who has permanently lost cardio-respiratory function is dead. The tests that are derived from these criteria are:
- absence of peripheral pulses;

- apnoea;
- no heart sounds.

In many textbooks another test is mentioned, namely that the individual should have fixed dilated pupils, but this test is not logically derived from the cardio-respiratory criteria and reflects brain function rather than cardio-respiratory function. As I mentioned in chapter 2, any qualified doctor in any location with the minimum of medical equipment can perform these tests and they need not be repeated. I have already argued in chapter 9 that these criteria (that is, the permanent loss of breathing and the permanent loss of the beating heart) can be used if the concept of death that I propose is adopted. There is no doubt that after a human being permanently loses the ability to maintain homeostasis there will be a period of time during which the heart will continue to beat and during which some form of breathing may occur although for a shorter time. When both spontaneous breathing has ceased and the heart has stopped beating (both events being assumed to be permanent) one can be confident that death has occurred although the conceptual point of death has occurred some time prior to the determination of death by these criteria. It follows from this that if the permanent loss of the ability to control homeostasis is accepted as death, then these criteria for death and the derived tests for death could be used within that concept without any change to these commonly applied criteria or tests. The proposed concept of death, therefore, does not require any change to these criteria or tests for death and they can be used, as before, to diagnose death confidently in the majority of cases.

Brainstem Death Criteria

According to the Medical Royal Colleges (Conference, 1976; Conference, 1979; Working Group, 1995), brain death is the death of the brainstem (for the purposes of this discussion, leave aside my previously stated objections to this statement) and can be recognised by establishing:
- coma with apnoea;
- absence of drug intoxication;
- absence of hypothermia;
- absence of hypoglycaemia (low blood sugar);
- absence of acidosis;
- absence of electrolyte imbalance.

The tests derived from these criteria are all tests of brainstem function and all brainstem reflexes should be absent:
- fixed, unreacting pupils with absent corneal response;

- no vestibulo-ocular reflexes, that is no eye movement after or during slow injection of 20mls of ice-cold water into each external auditory meatus in turn;
- no motor response to adequate stimuli within the cranial nerve area;
- no gag reflex or response to bronchial stimulation;
- no respiratory effort on stopping the ventilator and allowing the P_aCO_2 to rise to 6.7kPa.

In contrast to the cardio-respiratory criteria, these tests must be repeated, usually after some hours, and must be performed by a consultant or a doctor qualified for a minimum of 5 years. Since the individual on whom the tests are performed would be apnoeic and requiring ventilation, the tests can only be performed in selected areas within a hospital *e.g.* an Intensive Therapy Unit.

We can see from this brief description that there has been a considerable change in the operational conditions and requirements for the diagnosis of death (in the small number of cases in whom the cardio-respiratory criteria cannot be applied) as a result of the introduction of the brainstem death concept of death and its associated criteria and tests into the UK. What I must consider now are the criteria and tests that are logically derived from my proposed concept of death and then consider whether or not there would be any further operational changes in the diagnosis of death as a result of the adoption of my concept of death. The criteria that can be derived from the concept of death, that is the permanent loss of homeostasis are:

- coma;
- loss of control of temperature regulation;
- loss of control of fluid balance;
- loss of control of blood pressure.

Like the brainstem death criteria, there are exclusion criteria that must be met prior to the performance of any test. The purpose of these exclusion criteria is to exclude any remedial or temporary cause for the clinical condition of the individual and to establish a cause for the clinical state; all the exclusion criteria must be met prior to any tests being performed. The exclusion criteria are:

- exclusion of other causes of coma;
- exclusion of other causes of low body temperature;
- exclusion of other causes of diabetes insipidus;
- exclusion of other causes of hypotension.

Once these exclusion criteria have been satisfied, the tests for death under my proposed concept of death can be performed:

- tests for unresponsive coma:
    - demonstration of coma by tests at present used for brainstem death;
- measurement of body temperature:
    - demonstration of low body temperature;
    - demonstration of falling body temperature;
- measurement of urine output:
    - demonstration of large, continued and inappropriate urine volumes;
- measurement of blood pressure:
    - demonstration of low blood pressure;
    - demonstration of falling blood pressure.

While it may appear to a lay person that there are a very large number of tests with my proposed concept of death, this is a false impression. All the measurements in the list above are routinely performed in an Intensive Therapy Unit where an individual undergoing these tests is required to be placed in order that ventilation can be given since, like an individual undergoing brainstem death tests, an individual undergoing brain death tests under my proposed concept of death would be apnoeic. If the fact that the latter three tests are routinely performed in an ITU is considered, then there would be no significant increase or change in the operational requirements for the diagnosis of death under my suggested concept of death compared to the diagnosis of death under the brainstem death concept of death. It would merely be the case that more clinical data would need to be considered, compared to the data considered for the brainstem death criteria, before the diagnosis of death could be made.

Having said that there is no significant increase in tests required under my concept of death compared with the current UK brainstem death criteria, I must consider whether there would be changes at all in the tests required, that is whether there are tests required under the brainstem criteria of death that my proposed concept of death would not require. The answer to this question can be obtained by close inspection of the tests derived from the criteria and listed above. In the case of the brainstem criteria, the tests are concentrated on the functions (but not all the functions) of the brainstem. In contrast to this concentration on some of the functions of the brainstem, the tests derived from my proposed concept of death concentrate on the functions of the pituitary and hypothalamus and make no reference to, nor need any test of, the functions of the brainstem. It follows from this that the tests for brainstem function necessary under the brainstem death concept of death are superfluous to the requirements of my proposed concept of death. Therefore, while there would be no significant increase in the number of tests to be performed under my criteria, there would be a major change in the actual tests performed; all tests specified in the section on brainstem death would no longer be needed. Under the concept of death advocated in this monograph, it would *not* be necessary to test for fixed unreacting pupils with absent corneal response, for oculo-vestibular reflexes, for a motor response within the cranial nerve area, for a gag reflex or for lack of respiratory effort with an adequate P_aCO_2.

There is one other matter concerning the current brainstem death concept of death and my proposed concept of death that requires discussion. This matter is the question of any association between my proposed criteria for death and the currently used brainstem death criteria. In other words, could the currently used tests for brainstem death be used consistently with my homeostatic concept of death? There are two approaches to the answer to this question:

- to describe what happens in clinical practice;
- to argue on theoretical grounds.

Firstly, let me describe what happens in clinical practice when brain death is occurring in an individual in an ITU. The individual concerned will be apnoeic and will be ventilated; at some point the blood pressure will begin to rise and pulse rate fall as pressure on the brainstem produces hypotension in that region. This rise in blood pressure will continue for a variable time but, at some point, the blood pressure will plummet to an extremely low level, as brainstem function is lost. At, or about, this time the urine output rises inexorably and the body temperature of the individual begins to fall as pituitary and hypothalamic function fails. Thus, the criteria for brainstem death and homeostatic death would be satisfied when the time came for the tests to be performed. Under these circumstances, the tests for brainstem death could be used as indicators that not only has brainstem death occurred, but also homeostatic death has occurred since the two events (that is brainstem death and homeostatic death) are so closely linked in practice. It would be reasonable, therefore, to accept that the tests for brainstem death could be used consistently with the homeostatic concept of death if it is accepted that the brainstem death tests are only an indirect method of assessing the integrity of homeostasis under these circumstances.

The second approach to ascertaining whether or not the brainstem death tests could be used consistently with my homeostatic concept of death would be to explore the matter on a theoretical basis as opposed to the practical approach that has been discussed above. I have already discussed earlier in this chapter the fact that the tests for brainstem death (as used in the UK) play no part in the diagnosis of homeostatic death and that the tests for homeostatic death have no rôle to play in the diagnosis of brainstem death, but this bald statement needs to be discussed further. I intend to do this by means of an analogy. Let me examine two events, A and B, that are separated in time such that A always precedes B and B is always preceded by A, and which each have distinct and separate "markers" that indicate when each event has happened. Under ordinary circumstances, event A would occur and this occurrence of A could be detected by detection of the appropriately associated "markers". This would be followed, at some later time, by event B the occurrence of which would be detected by the markers for B. Since A always precedes B and B is always preceded by A, it follows that if the occurrence of event A was to be detected, it could be done either directly by detecting the markers for event A or, indirectly, by detecting the markers for event B. Let me now substitute the time of homeostatic death for event A, the tests for homeostatic death for the markers for event A, the time of brainstem death for event B and the tests for brainstem death for the markers for event B. It should be clear, from the analogy, that homeostatic death could either be detected directly using the tests for homeostatic death or indirectly using the tests for brainstem death. It would thus seem that the tests for brainstem death could be used consistently within the homeostatic concept of death. This conclusion depends, of course, on the conditions set out in the analogy and, in particular, the conditions that relate to the temporal association between events A and B. If it can be demonstrated that, in practice, the relationship between homeostatic death and brainstem death does not conform to the description of the temporal association between events A and B in the analogy, then my conclusion would not be correct, and the tests for brainstem death could not be used consistently within the concept of homeostatic death. I therefore need to discuss the possibility that event A is not always followed by event B and also the possibility that event B is not, in all cases, preceded by event A. In the case where event A is not followed by event B, it follows that since there has been no event B there will be no "markers" for event B. The detection of event A, therefore must rest entirely upon direct detection using only the "markers" for event A. Using the same substitutions for events A and B and their associated "markers" as before, it is clear that under the circumstances whereby event A is not followed by event B, homeostatic death would not be followed by brainstem death and that homeostatic death could be diagnosed only directly using the tests for homeostatic death that have been described earlier in this chapter. Under these circumstances, that is homeostatic death

Operational Changes as a Result of the Suggested Concept of Death   165

not followed by brainstem death, the tests for brainstem death would be negative, that is would not confirm the diagnosis of brainstem death; it follows from that that negative tests for brainstem death cannot exclude homeostatic death since homeostatic death may have occurred without brainstem death ensuing. I must now consider the circumstances in which event B is not always preceded by event A. Under these circumstances, the "markers" for event A would not be detected but the "markers" for event B would have been. It follows, therefore, that under these circumstances detection of event B could not be used, indirectly, to detect the previous occurrence of event A. If, again, we use the same substitutions for event A and B and their "markers", it should be obvious that should brainstem death occur without preceding homeostatic death, then the positive results of the brainstem death tests (confirming the diagnosis of brainstem death) could not be used to, indirectly, detect the presence of homeostatic death. The end result of the discussion of the two sets of circumstances, namely that event A may not be followed by event B in all cases, and that event B may not be preceded, in all cases, by event A is that the tests for brainstem death may not reliably indicate that homeostatic death has already occurred. Critical examination of the two concepts of brainstem death and homeostatic death and their associated tests, therefore, indicate that the tests for brainstem death cannot be used reliably to diagnose indirectly homeostatic death; the only reliable tests for homeostatic death are the direct ones, that is the tests derived from the criteria for homeostatic death. This conclusion, however, disregards the physiological fact that permanent loss of homeostasis always results in death of all other areas of the brain and, indeed, death of all the tissues in the organism (see chapter 8 for a deeper discussion) and brainstem death leads very quickly to permanent loss of control of homeostasis. It probably would be a much better analogy, then, if it was altered to accommodate these important facts. In that case, the analogy should be altered to the extent that event A is always, and without exception, followed by event B and event B is always and without exception preceded by event A. As a result of this alteration, it follows that if event B has not occurred, then event A has not occurred and the absence of "markers" for event B could be used to indicate with certainty, but indirectly, the non-occurrence of event A. It follows, with the same substitutions as before, that a negative test for brainstem death can be used to indirectly indicate the absence of homeostatic death. In summary, therefore, a negative test for brainstem death is a reliable indicator of the absence of homeostatic death and a positive test for brainstem death can be used reliably to demonstrate the presence of homeostatic death. It should be noted at this point that the end result of this argument does not match the end result of the first way of looking at the problem. If one examines clinical practice, the conclusion reached is that the tests for brainstem death could be used as an indirect indicator of homeostatic death.

The question to be addressed now is how the changes in the required tests could be introduced into the clinical setting in which they would be used. There would appear to be two ways in which this could be done, the first being the more intellectually rigorous and the second being more pragmatic. The first of these, the more intellectually rigorous of the two, would be to adopt my proposed concept of death with its derived criteria and tests and use it without reference to any other concept of brain death. In other words, my proposed concept of homeostatic death would be used in isolation and entirely separate from the current concept of brainstem death. The alternative position would be to amalgamate my proposed concept of homeostatic death with the present concept of brainstem death. This would not be as intellectually rigorous or as satisfying as the first option, but could be carried out. The tests for homeostatic death could be performed alongside the tests for brainstem death and both sets of tests recorded and this would require very little extra work. A difficulty would arise, however, when it came to the declaration of death since it would not be clear which concept of death was being used. If the brainstem death concept of death is being used, then there is no need to perform the tests for homeostatic death and if the homeostatic concept of death is the concept in use, then there is no need to perform the tests for brainstem death. This approach, namely combining the two sets of tests would only lead to intellectual confusion and the one thing that should be apparent from reading this monograph is that the concept of death needs clarity of thought.

I have already indicated that the present brainstem death tests could be accommodated within my suggested concept of death. I now intend to discuss the relationship between this proposed concept of death and the beating heart/breathing criteria for death. It may help if an analogy is used to illustrate my concept of death and the relationship between the beating heart/ breathing criteria and the brainstem concept of death. Let us imagine a house the outside surroundings of which represents life and the inside of which represents death. In order to pass from the state of being alive to the state of being dead, a person must enter the house by a door; the door represents the permanent loss of the ability to control homeostasis. Once the person concerned has passed through this door, the person takes some steps into the house; these steps represent the successive failures of different functions or systems. A feature of this analogy to be emphasised is the difference between death occurring and death being detected. Under my concept of death, death has occurred when the person has passed through the door, that is when homeostasis has been irretrievably lost, but death cannot be detected at this point for two reasons:

- there is an inescapable time lag between the control of homeostasis ceasing to exist permanently and any biochemical or physiological change of the type being used as tests for death being apparent in the human being so affected;
- once any such biochemical or physiological change has occurred, the change must reach a critical level before it can be detected by present biochemical or physiological tests.

For these reasons, the point at which death has occurred conceptually and the point at which death can be detected in practice is not one and the same point but are separated by a period of time. Within the analogy, although death has occurred conceptually when the person stepped through the door, death cannot be detected at this point but only at some later time after some steps into the house have been taken, that is when some function or system has failed and the failure can be detected. Now, since functions or systems fail at different times after death has occurred and tests for death depend upon the detection of such failures (for example the loss of heartbeat or breathing) to detect death, it follows that different tests using different functions or systems will detect death at different times. Within the analogy, this would mean that although death occurred conceptually (according to the concept of death that I advocate) when the human being passed through the door, death would not be detected until some steps into the house had been taken, the exact number of steps being dependent upon the tests used for death. For example, if the tests for death are the tests for the loss of control of homeostasis then death may be diagnosed after relatively few steps into the house whereas if the criteria of the loss of the beating heart and breathing are used then more steps would have been taken prior to death being diagnosed and if the criterion of putrefaction derived from yet another concept of death is used then even more steps would have been taken prior to the diagnosis of death being reached; if the criteria of brainstem death is used then the number of steps taken into the house would be only slightly greater than the number of steps taken if the criteria from my suggested concept of death had been used to determine death.

Therefore, using my suggested concept of death, death can be diagnosed using the criteria of the beating heart and breathing but the diagnosis of death will be reached later than it would have been reached if the criteria for homeostatic death had been used.

Public Policy Considerations

I have discussed, in the earlier part of this chapter, the practical considerations of the introduction of my proposed concept of homeostatic death but there are other problems that it would be prudent to bear in mind. For some people, death is signified by the absence of pulse and breathing and for these persons any standards, criteria and tests that use brain function to determine whether death has occurred are seriously in error. I have argued both earlier in this chapter and in chapter 10 that the commonly used tests for death, namely absence of pulse and breathing are consistent with the concept of homeostatic death and it would seem that the homeostatic concept of death has that advantage over the brainstem concept of death which cannot accommodate these two tests within it. The two tests of absence of pulse and breathing are, therefore, tests that can be used within the proposed concept of death rather than tests that must remain outside. While it may seem a straightforward matter to educate public opinion on this matter, I am not so sure of this. There has been a history of misuse of medical terms in the media even several years after the introduction of the concept of brainstem death (Frame, 1995). In addition, there has been misrepresentation of medical facts in a widely viewed television programme (Panorama, 1980). The programme questioned the validity of the criteria and the certainty of the tests but failed to explain that the exclusion criteria used before the brainstem tests are considered had been ignored. The patients considered in the programme had all recovered after extended periods of unconsciousness but, as was pointed out in many medical criticisms of the programme, none of those patients whose cases were examined had ever met the criteria required for the diagnosis of brainstem death (Luksza, Atherton, Jones, Dawes, Daniels and Bisasur, 1980). As a result of this programme, many potential organ transplant recipients did not receive organs as the organ donor rate fell (Bradley and Brooman, 1980). Under these circumstances of misrepresentation, I have no great hopes for rapid public education in this matter.

It is, perhaps, not surprising that there is some confusion in the minds of a non-medically qualified audience since there is no firm consensus about the meaning of the terms "brain death" and "brainstem death" within medicine itself. The Conference of Colleges (1979) argued that the diagnosis of brainstem death meant, "all functions of the brain have permanently and irreversibly ceased" since brainstem death was the physiological core of brain death and that the identification of brainstem death meant that the patient was dead. This statement differs from the statement from the same source in 1976 (Conference, 1976) in which the state of brainstem death was taken to be a very accurate predictor of death in the immediate future, and differs significantly from the most recent announcement from the Working Group of the Royal College of Physicians (1995). This latter group reviewed criteria for the diagnosis of brainstem death and no longer claimed that, when brainstem death is diagnosed, "all functions of the brain have permanently and irreversibly ceased" and suggested that the term "brainstem death" should be used in preference to the term "brain death" to avoid confusion. The same group also suggested "irreversible loss of the capacity for consciousness, combined with irreversible loss of the capacity to breathe" should be regarded as the definition of death. This is a surprising statement from this group who advocate that the criteria of death should be logically derived from explicitly formulated philosophical premises in view of the lack of a convincing theory of consciousness (Polkingthorne, 1994). Even Pallis, a strong supporter of the brainstem concept of death, concedes that there is no convincing theory of consciousness (Pallis, 1996), but argues for a pragmatic solution. All this activity from the Royal College of Physicians seems to indicate some confusion in the concept of brainstem death:

- Is it merely prognostic of death as they originally advocated in 1976?
- Does it represent death as they advocated in 1979?
- Is it logically derived from sound philosophical premises if one of the components of brainstem death, unconsciousness, has no underlying convincing theory?

With this amount of confusion inside the medical profession, it is no wonder that there is a degree of confusion outside the profession.

There is hope, however, that a well-argued position may prevail. The recent announcement from the Royal College of Physicians (1995) recognises that the criteria for death must be logically derived from explicitly formulated philosophical premises. This is exactly what I have attempted to do in this monograph. I would hope that such an approach, that is the development of criteria and tests for death from a sound philosophical premise, and the arguments employed throughout the monograph would permit serious consideration of the permanent loss of control of homeostasis as a concept of death that is both philosophically sound and useful in practice.

Future Developments

Medical technology is constantly advancing and challenging many of the accepted theories and treatments within the practice of medicine. It is appropriate to consider what effect possible advances may have on my suggested monograph that permanent loss of control of homeostasis entails death. What if, at some time in the future, a "chip" implant could replace spontaneous control of homeostasis?

There have been recorded in the literature two cases in which control of homeostasis has been permanently lost and in which such control of homeostasis has been supplied by external means; these cases have been discussed by Singer (1995). Both cases would seem, at first sight, to create insuperable problems for my suggested concept of death. How are we to view individuals under such circumstances? I shall put to one side the legal position of individuals in this clinical state and consider the philosophical responses to the problem. In terms of the currently accepted or advocated concepts of death, individuals such as the two described above should be viewed as being dead, since they fail to exhibit any signs of either brainstem or neocortical function. Those who hold to the beating heart/breathing concept of death would view such individuals as being alive until both functions had ceased. The greatest problem that these two cases pose, or at least appear to pose, is to the concept of death that I propose in this monograph, namely that permanent loss of control of homeostasis entails death. The easy solution to this problem would be to take the stance that the individuals concerned have permanently lost control of homeostasis and are, therefore, in terms of my proposed concept of death to be considered dead. However, let us suppose that instead of external support of homeostasis as was supplied to the two individuals under discussion, there could be internal support and that some form of "chip" could be inserted and that homeostasis could be controlled indefinitely. What should be the response under these circumstances when the individuals concerned would closely approximate the persistent vegetative state? Before trying to answer that question, let us consider another scenario. Let us consider not only that a "chip" can be inserted to control homeostasis but that this can be done prior to the failure of other areas of the brain. What we could have under these circumstances would be an individual who has homeostasis being controlled but who, at the same time, was able to walk, talk and otherwise conduct a normal life. What should our response be under these circumstances to the question of whether such an individual is alive or dead? The question being posed here is the one that has been posed to other concepts of death in the face of scientific and medical advance (see chapter one for a review of the history of death) and it is the same question that faced supporters of the beating heart/breathing criteria for death when heart transplants were first performed. Is the important thing the spontaneous function of the heart or does it matter that the function is supplied by a transplanted heart or even a totally artificial heart or stimulated by a cardiac pacemaker? I shall return to this question later in this chapter.

If we now return to the question of a "chip" replacing the spontaneous control of homeostasis, there are three immediate answers to this question:

- The first reply is to take the stance that there is permanent loss of control of homeostasis in the individuals who have been given the "chip" implant and that, under the terms of my proposed concept of death, such an individual should be viewed as being dead. However, it would be difficult to say that an individual who conducted his life in a normal manner should be viewed as dead when I have already argued that an individual in the locked-in syndrome should be viewed as alive, as indeed all such individuals are viewed at present.
- The second reply is to say that there is permanent loss of spontaneous control of homeostasis but that there is still control of homeostasis by some means and, accordingly, the individual in this state should be viewed as being alive. Such a reply would seem to satisfy the common-sense approach that an individual who is walking, talking and living life normally should be viewed as alive.
- The third reply would be to argue that spontaneous control of homeostasis has been lost and whilst control of homeostasis is being maintained by artificial means, a new category of individuals has been created and that another term, that is neither "dead" nor "alive", should be applied to them. I think that this approach to the problem is counterintuitive and an affront to reason and would create unnecessary philosophical and legal muddle.

I would like to return to the second suggestion and explore it in greater depth. I have suggested there the case of an individual who has permanently lost spontaneous control of homeostasis but who has been given a "chip" capable of controlling homeostasis is to be viewed as alive.

This would seem, *prima facie*, to present difficulties for my suggested monograph that permanent loss of control of homeostasis entails death. The difficulties alluded to here are the same as the difficulties already mentioned earlier in this section in relation to the beating heart/breathing criteria for death and the use of cardiac transplants and cardiac pacemakers. In the latter case there is no spontaneous cardiac function—but the heart is "driven" by the pacemaker and in the former case, the heart is not the original heart of the patient. Is spontaneity of function all-important or do we accept non-spontaneity of function as having the same importance as spontaneity of the same function? Society had no moral difficulty with this question inasmuch as those individuals who had received a transplanted heart were viewed unanimously as being alive. While moral disquiet was associated with the question of cardiac transplantation, it was the act of transplantation that generated the disquiet not the status of the transplant recipient. To my knowledge, there has been no philosophical argument put forward to suggest that cardiac transplant recipients should be regarded as anything other than alive. It would seem, from these two points, that spontaneity of function is not important in this matter; an individual should be viewed as alive irrespective of the spontaneity or non-spontaneity of cardiac function, or in this case, of control of homeostasis. Allow me to examine this topic from another perspective. I have viewed the concept of life along the lines indicated by Schrödinger (1994), namely that life is the ability to control entropy and, in the human, the ability to control homeostasis. However, it is Schrödinger's view that such a concept of life should apply to all life and not merely to human beings and with this I am in complete agreement. With this idea that this concept of life (and death) should be applicable to all life, let us examine how other forms of life control entropy and, in particular, let us look at the animals classified as poikilothermic. These animals are not able to control body temperature by an internal mechanism and, in order to keep body temperature within the range in which they can live, they are required to move into warm or cool areas as the need arises. If such an animal is prevented from moving into the appropriate temperature range, it will eventually die. Let us now consider the scenario in which such an animal is unable to move (the reason for the immobility is not relevant to my argument) and depends upon being moved into an area of appropriate temperature range by an external force, for example being wheeled into such areas by a keeper of some description, but is otherwise able to lead a normal life. Under these circumstances, it could be said that such an animal is dependent upon external control of its homeostasis; nevertheless it would continue to be viewed as alive. I suggest that this scenario does not differ in its important aspects from the scenario described in the second paragraph above in which a human being leads a normal life despite spontaneous control of homeostasis being permanently lost and a "chip" supplying the necessary control. The human being under these circumstances should be classified as alive.

It should be borne in mind that this discussion about the problems arising from the insertion of a "chip" capable of controlling homeostasis in a human being is purely academic for two reasons:

- There is no such "chip" at present and it is extremely unlikely that one could be developed in the foreseeable future. While the discussion concerning the implantation of such a "chip" is important philosophically, it should not be assumed that such discussion implies that such a procedure is even remotely possible.
- The scenario in which a "chip" controlling homeostasis could be inserted into a human being prior to failure of the control of homeostasis with the result that such a human being could thereafter lead a normal life presupposes that the control of homeostasis is lost while the other physiological systems are intact and operating normally. This supposition is, in general, incorrect since in the ordinary course of events, it is damage to and failure of other physiological systems that results in the loss of control of homeostasis; return of the control of homeostasis by the implanting of a "chip" would not return function to the other physiological systems damaged and would not, in all probability, result in the return of the control of homeostasis since the other physiological systems would be needed for control of homeostasis to be effected. In practical terms, therefore, the implantation of such a "chip" would not result in a human being leading a normal life.

However, both these reasons for considering that a "chip" replacing the spontaneous control of homeostasis is academic are contingent reasons and it is possible to consider that:

- Such a chip could be made in the future if one considers the advances made in the appropriate technology that have occurred in recent years.
- Implantation of such a chip may become possible. Consider the implantation of an artificial cochlea allowing hearing in previously deaf individuals, the implantation of phrenic nerve stimulators to allow "breathing" without an external ventilator in the case of individuals with a complete cervical spinal injury that made spontaneous breathing impossible or the implantation of sacral nerve stimulators to allow

individuals with spinal cord damage control over their own denervated bladder that previously was outwith their control; all these procedures were considered impossible a few years ago.
- There are primary disturbances of the hypothalamus (the area of brain concerned with control of homeostasis) and homeostatic function such that the control of homeostasis may be disturbed (or lost in severe instances). Examples of such primary disturbances would be:
  (1) Familial dysautonomia or the Riley-Day syndrome. This is inherited as an autosomal recessive trait and is a rare disease of infancy and childhood. Manifestations include excessive perspiration, peripheral vascular disturbances, postural hypotension and erratic temperature control.
  (2) The Fröhlich or adrenogential syndrome. This was the first hypothalamic syndrome to be described. It usually occurs in boys and is characterised by disturbances of fat metabolism together with sexual underdevelopment.

There are, therefore, well-established primary disturbances of hypothalamic function indicating that control of homeostasis may be disturbed and potentially lost as a primary event and not necessarily lost as described as a secondary event as described above. It seems, therefore, that the two reasons given earlier in this section for considering that the use of a "chip" to control homeostasis was an academic discussion are merely contingent reasons and that there is no logical reason why such reasons must prevail in all future cases. It may well become possible to devise and implant a "chip" to control homeostasis in those individuals in whom the spontaneous control of homeostasis is failing and in whom there is no failure of the peripheral components organs of homeostasis. Under these circumstances, such an individual would be viewed as being alive.

Having argued that "chip" implantation to allow control of homeostasis does not pose a problem for my proposal that permanent loss of control of homeostasis entails death, there does remain the potential problem of death after the implantation of such a "chip". By this I mean the potential problem of how individuals with such a "chip" controlling homeostasis come to die. It could be argued that they must die because of failure of part of or the whole of another physiological system. At first sight, this would seem to be the case. Such individuals (those with "chip" implants), it would seem, will need to die from diseases or disorders of other physiological systems (for example, heart failure, respiratory failure or a major stroke) since failure of control of homeostasis is unlikely to occur in the presence of the "chip" implant. The logical conclusion of such an argument, if accepted, would mean that death had been transferred to somewhere else in the body, in other words the locus of death would not be the hypothalamus but some other organ in some other physiological system and death would no longer be entailed by the permanent loss of control of homeostasis. This argument, however, is very similar to the argument against my monograph that I discussed in chapter 8; in that chapter I argued against the idea that anything that contributed toward homeostasis should count toward homeostasis. In chapter 8, the contention was that all components of homeostasis should count in the same way as homeostasis and I argued that the control of homeostasis was of far greater importance than any individual component of the systems controlled. In the case of the "chip" insertion, similar arguments are being raised to allow the locus of death to be transferred from the control of homeostasis to some other organ in some other physiological system, for example to the heart. However, if we examine the arguments I used in chapter 8, we find that they are applicable in this case. Consider for a moment what happens when the respiratory system begins to fail and oxygen and carbon dioxide cannot be exchanged in the quantities required by metabolism. Under these circumstances, the central control of homeostasis causes the respiratory rate to increase in an attempt to increase the exchange of gases and the renal excretion of acidic compounds is increased to compensate for the increase in plasma acidity caused by the retention of (or reduced ability to excrete) carbon dioxide. In other words, the increasing failure of one organ or system is compensated for by mechanisms brought into play and controlled by the central control of homeostasis. As the failure of the respiratory system progresses, there will come a time when the inability to exchange oxygen and carbon dioxide cannot be compensated for by the mechanisms I have outlined above and homeostasis cannot be maintained; in other words, the control of homeostasis has failed. At this point other physiological systems will begin to fail as the necessary requirements for their continued functioning are not maintained, that is there is no oxygen being supplied and the acidity of the fluids surrounding the cells of the organs that constitute the physiological system exceeds the level at which the cells can exist. The whole organism will then cease to function as a whole and, indeed, as I argued in chapter 8, the organism ceases to function as a whole when control of homeostasis has been permanently lost. I suggest that it does not matter whether this control of homeostasis is supplied spontaneously or by a "chip" implanted some time earlier. The implanted "chip" must, of necessity, control homeostasis within the same limits as spontaneous control of homeostasis for the very good and insurmountable reason that those limits are the limits within which the cells and organs of the body are able to survive and function. Therefore, at the point at which spontaneous control of homeostasis would fail to control homeostasis the implanted "chip" would also fail to control homeostasis. Therefore, the scenario that I have described above in which the respiratory system failed progressively would be handled in exactly the same way by spontaneous control of homeostasis and an implanted "chip". The conclusion is, therefore, that death is entailed by loss of control of homeostasis however that is supplied (spontaneously or by an implanted "chip").

From this line of argument it can be seen that my proposed monograph that permanent loss of control of homeostasis entails death of the organism is a robust monograph and is unlikely to be superseded by advances in medical technology.

Summary

In this chapter I have outlined the changes that would be entailed by the adoption of my proposed monograph that death is entailed by the permanent loss of control of homeostasis; these are minimal and do not constitute a practical bar to the adoption of the concept of death proposed in my monograph. I have also argued that advances in medical technology do not pose an insuperable problem to my proposed concept of death and that it would be applicable under circumstances that are barely imaginable at the present time.

References

Bradley, B.A. and Brooman, P.M. (1980), "Panorama's lost transplants", *Lancet*, vol. ii, pp. 1258-1259.
Conference of the Medical Royal Colleges and their Faculties in the UK (1976), "Diagnosis of death", *Brit. Med. J.,* vol. ii, pp. 1187-1188.
Conference of the Medical Royal Colleges and their Faculties in the UK (1979), "Diagnosis of death", *Brit. Med. J.,* vol. i, p. 3320.
Frame, L. (1995), "My little girl dies three times a week", *The Sun*, March 8, pp. 1-2.
Luksza, A.R., Atherton, S.T., Jones, E.S., Dawes, P., Daniels, J.A. and Bisasur, P. (1980), "Transplants—are the donors really dead?", *Brit. Med. J.,* pp. 281:1140.
Pallis, C. (1996), "Brain stem death—In response", *J. R. Coll. Physicians London,* vol. 30(1), pp. 88-89.
Panorama. (1980), BBC Television.
Polkingthorne, J. (1974), *Science and Christian belief*, S.P.C.K., London, p. 27.

Schrödinger, E. (1944), *What is life?*, Cambridge Univ. Press, Cambridge, (reprint 1992), pp. 67-75.

Singer, P. (1995), *Rethinking life and death*, Oxford Univ. Press, Melbourne, pp. 9-16.

Working Group of the Royal College of Physicians. (1995), "Criteria for the diagnosis of brain stem death", *J. R. Coll. Physicians London*, vol. 29, pp. 381-382.

Index

abnormal brain states, 39, 40, 49, 50, 85
  comparison with locked-in sysndrome, 42
anencephalic, 22, 65, 67, 84, 87, 103, 105
  survivors, 84
anencephaly, 84, 87
anoxia, 23, 144
apallic syndrome, 41
apnoea, 22, 26, 32, 33, 50, 160
artificial ventilation, 9, 19, 33, 45, 46, 47, 54, 81

beating heart, 11, 32, 51, 92, 130, 131, 132, 142, 144, 145, 156, 159, 160, 166, 167, 168, 170, 172
  argument against as test for death, 144
biological concept of death
  practical arguments, 116
blood gas levels, 97
bodily integrity, 24, 79, 81, 85, 100, 107, 110, 115, 119, 121, 141, 142, 147, 159
boundaries of life, 109
brain dead, 7, 10, 17, 19, 24, 33, 36, 37, 39, 77, 79, 87, 88
brain death, 6, 9, 11, 12, 13, 15, 17, 18, 19, 20, 21, 22, 23, 24, 25, 26, 27, 29, 30, 31, 35, 36, 37, 41, 42, 43, 45, 46, 47, 48, 49, 50, 51, 53, 54, 55, 56, 73, 74, 75, 76, 78, 79, 84, 85, 86, 87, 88, 105, 110, 131, 132, 135, 136, 137, 139, 140, 141, 142, 143, 144, 145, 146, 160, 162, 163, 166, 169
  current concepts, 25
  definition of, 42
  first case, 6
  Harvard criteria, 18
  necessary for death, 135
  operational significance, 29
  predictive value, 20, 22
  recognition, 18
  sufficient for death, 140
  variation in concept, 18
  versions of, 24
brainstem death, 14, 19, 24, 25, 26, 27, 29, 30, 32, 34, 35, 42, 46, 48, 49, 54, 55, 76, 78, 79, 81, 85, 86, 136, 146, 159, 161, 162, 163, 166, 167, 168, 169
  and changes in blood pressure, 77
  and death of other areas of brain, 28
  and persisting oesophageal function, 77
  and pituitary function, 77
  "broad" definition, 78
  definition of, 42
  haemodynamic responses, 28
  "narrow" definition, 78
  not total cessation of all functions of brainstem, 77
  oesophageal activity, 28
  partial, 48
  pituitary gland, 28
  predictive value, 19
brainstem reflexes, 26, 32, 160

breathing, 1, 2, 7, 10, 11, 21, 22, 23, 30, 31, 32, 42, 46, 49, 50, 51, 54, 78, 81, 82, 84, 85, 92, 93, 113, 116, 130, 131, 138, 139, 140, 142, 144, 145, 149, 150, 156, 159, 160, 166, 167, 168, 170, 172, 174
  comparison with ventilation, 49
  in relation to moral status, 49
  comparison with beating heart, 51

capacity for personal experience, 29, 76
capacity for social interaction, 29, 31, 61, 68, 76, 83
capacity to appreciate pain, 21
cardiac by-pass, 93
cardiac pacemaker, 93
central heating system
  analogy with brain and other altered brain states, 53
cerebral death, 25, 41, 42, 43, 48
coma, 2, 9, 12, 18, 26, 32, 35, 36, 41, 42, 43, 65, 73, 84, 85, 87, 105, 118, 160, 161, 162
  definition of, 40
concept of death, 5, 11, 22, 24, 25, 26, 27, 29, 30, 31, 32, 33, 34, 35, 37, 50, 60, 61, 62, 64, 65, 66, 68, 70, 72, 73, 78, 79, 82, 83, 84, 85, 86, ,88, 92, 101, 103, 106, 107, 108, 110, 112, 113, 115, 116, 117, 119, 121, 133, 136, 137, 138, 140, 141, 142, 145, 147, 159, 160, 161, 162, 163, 166, 167, 168, 169, 170, 171, 176
  biological, 107, 115
  biological terms, 110
  commonality of, 112
  esoteric, 60
  in relation to different brain states, 75
  irreversible loss of soul, 62
  loss of capacity for bodily integration, 64
  loss of capacity for consciousness and social interaction, 65
  loss of consciousness, 66
  loss of flow of vital fluids, 63
  loss of personal identity, 67
  loss of rationality, 66
  loss of social interaction, 68
  non-biological terms, 110
  operational changes as a result of, 159
  philosophical, 114
  reasons for adopting a, 61
  religious, 114
  theoretical arguments, 109
  uniform, 102
consciousness, 9, 10, 20, 21, 24, 25, 27, 29, 40, 41, 42, 43, 47, 48, 52, 65, 66, 68, 69, 70, 73, 76, 78, 79, 80, 81, 82, 84, 110, 114, 115, 117, 118, 147, 169
  altered level of, 40
  problems with animals, 117
control of homeostasis, 51, 97, 100, 101, 103, 107, 121, 130, 136, 137, 139, 141, 148, 151, 152, 153, 154, 155, 157, 165, 170, 171, 172, 173, 174
  permanent loss of, 107
corneal reflex, 32
criteria for death, 60
  changes in, 12
  esoteric, 60
  free-floating, 60
  infallibility, 93

death
  analogy with train stopping, 155
  common conception of, 39
  conceptual point of, 147
  definition of, 8, 9
  departure of soul, 29
  diagnosis, 1
  discovery of point of, 17
  equivocal meaning, 70
  erroneous diagnosis, 3
  failure of whole organism, 148
  in antiquity, 1
  insensitivity of tests, 7
  metaphorical, 116
  moment of lethal insult, 151
  moment of manifestations of loss of homeostasis, 152
  multiple, 24
  neocortical, 11
  predictive value for, 142
  redefinition of, 9
  selection of brain as vital, 19
  selection of point of, 17
  tests for, 5
  time at which it can be said to have occurred, 147
  time at which it occurs, 147
  time at which loss of homeostasis has occurred, 153
  time of, 147
  time of which it can be said that loss of homeostasis has occurred, 154
  traditional tests for, 10
  uncertainty of diagnosis, 3, 4, 7
  whole brain criteria, 11
delirium, 40
dementia
  total, 41
diagnosis of death
  brainstem criteria, 160
  cardiorespiratory criteria, 159
  changes in tests with new concept of death, 162
  current UK criteria, 159
  suggested criteria from new concept of death, 161
  tests for death from the new concept of death, 162

EEG, 8
electroencephalogram, 8, 26
entropy, 6, 90, 91, 98, 99, 140, 172
  analogy with library, 91
  definition, 90

failure of the whole organism
  loss of integration, 148
failure of the whole organism
  material destruction, 148
  wholesale loss of function, 148
fluid balance, 42, 43, 44, 50, 97, 119, 124, 161

gag response, 32

Harvard criteria. *See* brain death
higher functions, 10, 24, 70, 72, 73
"higher function" concept of death
  general criticism of, 69
Hippocrates, 2
historical review, 1
homeostasis, 28, 42, 43, 46, 50, 56, 77, 78, 79, 82, 83, 86, 90, 92, 95, 96, 97, 98, 99, 100, 101, 102, 103, 104, 107, 119, 121, 126, 129, 135, 136, 137, 138, 139, 141, 144, 146, 147, 148,

151, 152, 153, 154, 155, 157,
160, 161, 163, 165, 166, 167,
170, 171, 172, 173, 174, 176
extraterrestrial life, 99
physiological importance of, 51
uniquely lost in brain death, 50
homoiothermic animals, 95
human being, 8, 25, 27, 54, 56,
62, 63, 65, 66, 67, 68, 70, 71,
76, 78, 79, 80, 81, 82, 84, 85,
86, 89, 90, 91, 93, 94, 98, 99,
102, 104, 107, 110, 112, 114,
126, 128, 129, 130, 131, 135,
136, 137, 138, 141, 143, 144,
145, 147, 149, 150, 156, 160,
167, 173
  as mammals, 102
  special case, 103
  value of, 103
human personhood, 25, 36
hyperthermia, 97
hypothermia, 14, 46, 97, 160

individual identity, 25
internal milieu, 92
irreplaceability, 20, 22

life
  necessary and sufficient conditions, 89
  Schrodinger's suggestion, 90
  seat of, 1
  sufficient conditions, 99
  suspension, 2
  what is, 90
LIS. *See* Locked-in syndrome
living organism, 94, 95, 100, 104,
living things
  common features, 98
  properties of, 94

locked-in syndrome, 41, 43, 45,
48, 49, 51, 54, 55, 81, 85, 136,
171
  communication in, 80
loss of sentience, 20, 21
low entropy state, 90, 98, 141

maximum entropy, 90, 91
Medical Royal Colleges. *See* Report
mutism, 41

nature of man, 25, 60
neocortical death,, 26, 27, 28, 29,
30, 35, 37, 41, 42, 43, 48, 70,
74, 76, 79, 80, 82, 84, 85, 86,
87, 88
  and personhood, 70
  legal death of the person, 76
nervous system
  integration, 7
not living
  two classes of, 94

organism
  as a whole, 6

permanent loss of consciousness,
10, 21, 27, 68, 69, 71, 76, 79,
81, 84, 117
permanent unconsciousness, 21,
42, 46, 48, 67, 78, 79, 118
persistent vegetative state, 21, 29,
32, 33, 39, 41, 43, 51, 54, 55,
56, 67, 79, 80, 82, 84, 86, 103,
118, 135, 136, 170
  maintenance of, 79
  neuropathological basis of, 41
  recovery from, 118
  terms synonymous with, 43
  Tony Bland, 80

person, 15, 25, 28, 30, 34, 40, 43, 45, 49, 54, 62, 64, 66, 68, 69, 70, 71, 72, 76, 79, 84, 93, 96, 105, 154, 162, 166, 167
personal existence, 1, 6
poikilothermic animals, 95
President's Commission. *See* Report
proposed concept of death
 "chip" implant, 171
 criteria for death, 161
 future developments, 170
 public policy considerations, 168
 tests for death, 162
psychological continuity, 29, 67, 82
pupillary response to light, 32
putrefaction, 4, 149, 150, 156, 167
 as sign of death, 3
PVS. *See* persistent vegetative state

Quinlan, 25, 36

Report
 Harvard Medical School, 18, 26
 Medical Royal Colleges (1976), 18
 Medical Royal Colleges (1979), 19
 President's Commission, 18
 University of Minnesota, 26
respiration
 tests for, 5
resuscitation, 4, 6, 7, 8, 13, 14, 15, 49, 93
rigor mortis, 5

single-cell organisms to human beings, 100
stethoscope, 6
suspended animation.4, 7, 8, 12, 16
system
 devaluation of components of, 130
 loss of control of, 131, 132
 multiple, 128
 value of, 121
 value of components, 121

tests for death
 brainstem death v new concept of death, 166
 changes in, 12
 electrical stimulation, 6
 infallibility of, 92
thermodynamic equilibrium, 90
trance, 4
transplant, 8, 17, 18, 23, 131, 168, 172
transplantation, 8, 9, 17, 20, 52, 172
treatment
 discontinuation, 17

unconsciousness, 21, 43, 46, 48, 50, 67, 69, 93, 118, 168, 169

vegetative state, 40
ventilator, 93
vestibulo-ocular reflex, 32
vital principle, 5

Western religions, 108
whole brain death, 25, 26, 27, 29, 35, 75, 76, 77, 85, 135, 136, 137, 141, 143